BREATHE SMARTER

RUN STRONGER

BREATHWORK TO TRANSFORM YOUR RUNNING

BREATHE SMARTER

RUN STRONGER

DAVID 'JACKO' JACKSON

BLOOMSBURY SPORT
Bloomsbury Publishing Plc
50 Bedford Square, London, WC1B 3DP, UK
Bloomsbury Publishing Ireland Limited,
29 Earlsfort Terrace, Dublin 2, D02 AY28, Ireland

BLOOMSBURY, BLOOMSBURY SPORT and the
Diana logo are trademarks of Bloomsbury Publishing Plc

First published in Great Britain 2026

Copyright © David Jackson, 2026

David Jackson has asserted his right under the Copyright,
Designs and Patents Act, 1988, to be identified as Author of this work

For legal purposes the Acknowledgements on p. 280 constitute an extension of this copyright page

All rights reserved. No part of this publication may be: i) reproduced or transmitted in any form, electronic or mechanical, including photocopying, recording or by means of any information storage or retrieval system without prior permission in writing from the publishers; or ii) used or reproduced in any way for the training, development or operation of artificial intelligence (AI) technologies, including generative AI technologies. The rights holders expressly reserve this publication from the text and data mining exception as per Article 4(3) of the Digital Single Market Directive (EU) 2019/790

Bloomsbury Publishing Plc does not have any control over, or responsibility for, any third-party websites referred to or in this book. All internet addresses given in this book were correct at the time of going to press. The author and publisher regret any inconvenience caused if addresses have changed or sites have ceased to exist, but can accept no responsibility for any such changes

A catalogue record for this book is available from the British Library

Library of Congress Cataloguing-in-Publication data has been applied for

ISBN: PB: 978-1-3994-2311-3; ePDF: 978-1-3994-2312-0; eBook 978-1-3994-2310-6

2 4 6 8 10 9 7 5 3 1

Typeset in IBM Plex Serif by Lumina Datamatics Ltd
Printed and bound in Great Britain by Clays Ltd, Elcograf S.p.A

Bloomsbury Publishing Plc makes every effort to ensure that the papers used in the manufacture of our books are natural, recyclable products made from wood grown in well-managed forests. Our manufacturing processes conform to the environmental regulations of the country of origin.

To find out more about our authors and books visit www.bloomsbury.com
and sign up for our newsletters
For product safety related questions contact productsafety@bloomsbury.com

This book is in memory of my father who
taught me how to be passionate about
the things we feel called to care about,
and who always believed in me.

Contents

Foreword by Patrick McKeown	9
Prologue	13
Introduction	16
My Story – Brain injury to breathing	20
1. What is breathing?	25
2. Smarter breathing	31
3. Why breathing has been overlooked, and why it's not your fault	45
4. What's the most important thing for runners?	58
5. Which hole in your face? The nose v mouth debate	81
6. Shut your mouth, lose your ego and train your airway	96
7. Breathing assessments	115
8. Unlock the power of your diaphragm	139
9. More mobility and less pain	164
10. More efficient with less oxygen	185
11. When the nose isn't enough	202
12. Recovery is a skill	214

13. Integrating into training and races	230
14. The golden rules	257
Breathe Smarter, Run Stronger checklist	273
References	274
Acknowledgements	280
Index	281

Foreword by Patrick McKeown

I believe that breathing training in sport will become a dominant focus within the next two to five years. Telling someone to 'take a few deep breaths' will be a thing of the past. Breathing training will become precise and individual, aligned with specific performance goals, and grounded in solid science. It will evolve from generic advice into tailored protocols that optimise endurance, speed, strength, recovery and mental clarity.

David Jackson is one of our most gifted Oxygen Advantage Master Instructors. In this book, 'Jacko' has created a thorough and highly practical guide to breathing for running. Drawing on his experience as a professional rugby player, his recovery from brain injury using breathing as a central tool, his interviews with leading experts in breathing training for sport and running performance, he brings together essential knowledge in a clear and accessible way.

Breathing training has made remarkable inroads since I began working in this field in 2002. At that time, it was viewed as left of field. Today, nasal breathing during exercise is a hot topic, and nasal breathing during sleep is even hotter. There is so much potential in the breath. Imagine simple tools that can be woven into everyday training and daily life to improve oxygenation, balance the nervous system, enhance resilience, open the airways, improve movement, delay lactic acid and fatigue, and train focus and concentration. For recreational runners, these benefits mean greater enjoyment, easier breathing and faster recovery. For elite athletes, breathing training offers a genuine competitive advantage.

There is nothing complicated about using the breath. After all, there are only a few ways we can change it to create different outcomes. In essence, we breathe in and we breathe out. What we do with this simple act can place the body and mind under severe stress, or it can bring deep relaxation, and everything in between.

We can choose to breathe faster or slower, take fuller breaths or breathe so lightly that only a wisp of air enters the lungs. We can breathe through the nose or the mouth, use the chest muscles more or rely primarily on the diaphragm, and we can hold the breath after inhaling or after exhaling. We might hold after inhaling for a few seconds, or exhale and sprint while holding the breath for 40m or more. Manipulating the breath to achieve a desired effect can be done at rest or during movement.

This practical range of breathing options, when used deliberately, can bring meaningful benefits to running. This book explores how targeted breathing methods can challenge old assumptions and turn the breath into a practical, trainable tool for runners.

I am in no doubt that this book is a disruptor for running. It will change how athletes approach training and competition. It will spark important conversations and influence progress in the sport for years to come.

Physical training alone does not train breathing. Running is usually practised with the mouth open, and this does not place sufficient load on the respiratory system to create adaptation. As every athlete knows, if you want to train something, you must add a specific load. Breathlessness is not simply a by-product of movement. It reflects the function of the respiratory system and needs to be targeted through breathwork.

Techniques such as nasal breathing during runs improve blood flow, oxygen delivery and oxygen utilisation. They also increase tolerance to carbon dioxide, helping the body become more efficient with each breath. Breathing is not only about performance. It also supports health. Nasal breathing during exercise boosts circulation to vital organs such as the heart and brain and helps with recovery.

To appreciate the power of nasal breathing for running, consider this example. In June 2024, Ihor Verys became the first finisher at the Barkley Marathons, one of the toughest race events in the world. Brutal is a more apt description! Since the race began in 1986, only around 20 runners have managed to complete all five loops, roughly 100 miles, within the 60-hour time limit. Verys openly credited his success to nasal breathing. He explained that other runners were unsettled to see him moving with controlled breathing, showing no outward sign of struggle. His body had been trained to sustain hard effort with reduced ventilation.

When it comes to running, it is also important that the mind does not get in the way. Otherwise, it can impose limits and sabotage performance. When the feeling of air hunger is strong and the breathing becomes heavy, the athlete's response to that sensation often determines whether they can keep going. The aim is to help an athlete do more with less by improving tolerance to carbon dioxide so there is no need to breathe so much air, and by training the brain to remain composed in the presence of breathlessness.

Mental willpower is a central feature of any sport, including running. How do you train the brain to hold attention on the task at hand, to stop overthinking, and to allow the athlete to perform with every cell of their body, fully present in a state of flow? Where is the mind of the runner during the run?

Do they have their attention on the breath, in the body, or in the moment? Or are they thinking about something other than what they are doing, going through the motions as it were. Doing one thing but thinking about something else. How can you expect optimal performance if you don't have your attention on the doing?

And the benefits here are that the practice during running carries into your everyday life, and the practice during your everyday life carries into running. In an age of distraction and stolen focus, it is time that we take this back. Otherwise it is to the detriment of our success, contentment and happiness. Running is not only training for the body. It is an opportune time to train the breath and, perhaps more importantly, to train the mind.

Breathing can place a hermetic stress on the body, causing positive adaptations that improve sports performance. Controlled breath-holds after exhalation lower blood oxygen, raise carbon dioxide, and create a strong air hunger.

I saw this clearly when working with Notre Dame athletes, all competing in track and field, mainly the 400m. Their training included a simple yet demanding protocol. They would sprint 360m at race pace, and just as fatigue began to take hold, they would exhale and hold the breath all the way to the finish line. The athlete learns to maintain form when the pressure is at its highest and to stay composed when it is most challenging.

Breathing practices are not only about pushing limits. Recovery is now understood as essential for performance, and the breath is a direct way to support it. Breathing exercises can calm the nervous system, improve sleep quality and sharpen focus, all of which play a central role in how an athlete performs during training and competition.

You might wonder why, if breathing can do all this, you have not heard more about it before. That is a fair question. The simplicity of breathing may be one reason. Exercise physiologists are typically not trained in breathing, and most doctors are not either. Breathing science in the context of exercise is only now beginning to catch up, years behind what instructors have observed in the field.

This book presents a practical framework for applying breathing principles to running. It emphasises that breathing interventions must be tailored to the individual runner. One single approach does not fit all. The aim is to make breathing an automatic part of running that supports performance, recovery, and overall well-being.

Jacko's book is not only a guide to running. It is a guide to living well through breath. When used consistently, these practices can unlock easier pace, more enjoyable runs, better recovery and a deeper sense of flow.

Patrick McKeown
Author of *The Oxygen Advantage*

Prologue

As usual we're running late. We pull up into the car park and take a final sip of a double espresso, which seems a little risky because it's 8:58 a.m. and parkrun is due to start in two minutes. We rush out of the car and see the more organised runners gathered together near the start line. It's the first time we've done this particular parkrun in Sheffield, so it would have been sensible to have turned up with enough time to hear the race briefing, but anyone who knows me and Catherine, my wife, knows that turning up on time can be a bit of a struggle.

Missing the race briefing wasn't an issue – it's not like you have to navigate in a parkrun, like you do in the mountains. I was never going to be right at the front; my personal best (PB) at this point was 20:20, so I could just follow the people ahead. I'm relieved we at least got to catch our breath, having sprinted from the car park to the start line. With a strong taste of the last-minute coffee still in the back of my throat, I felt slightly sick, but as the starter said 'go', I just put my head down as usual and set off at what was a pretty fast pace for me.

At this stage in my running journey, my training and goals consisted of turning up to a parkrun slightly late, where rushing to the start line was essentially the warm-up. Then just go as hard as I can and see if I can break my PB. That horrible metallic taste in my mouth, teeth aching at the end of the sprint finish as I collapse over the finish line was a familiar feeling that I equated to 'giving it everything'. Sometimes the bad combination of being late and drinking coffee within one minute of starting and pushing myself so hard meant I was actually sick after crossing the finishing line.

Today, though, was different. I had a new technique I was testing out about the importance of breathing. Something I'd completely overlooked during my professional rugby career and never considered before taking up running. For the last four weeks I'd been learning about how the way you breathe can make a difference to the way you get oxygen into your lungs, into your blood and to your muscles. It made sense to me once I understood some of the basic physiology and, in fact, I felt a bit stupid that I'd never considered it before. But I wasn't alone. Breathing wasn't something anyone was trying to get better at, we were just trying to run faster.

I'd not been practising long; I wasn't even sure if what I was doing was right, but I was keen to give it a go this morning. Although, I was a little sceptical because breathing is automatic, right? And it's so simple, could it really make a difference?

I tried to hang on to those ahead of me who were likely far better runners than me. As I started to struggle to keep up with their pace, my breathing started to become very fast and heavy. *Oh yeah, try and control it*, I thought to myself. I started to implement what I'd been learning about and settled into a rhythm. Rather than focusing on the runners ahead of me, I focused on my breathing.

As I approached the end, I actually felt really good and was keen to empty the tank as usual. The problem I had was that I didn't know the course. We approached what turned out to be the final bend and about 20m ahead was the finish line. I couldn't believe it. No sprint finish. I crossed the line, stopped my watch but didn't dare look at the time. Usually, I'd have the parkrun volunteers shouting at me to 'stay in line' as I'd peel myself off the floor, having collapsed over the finish line. But this week I felt like I'd not really tried that hard. I'd not pushed myself and was actually pretty gutted.

I waited a minute or so and clapped the other runners in, including Catherine. 'How did you get on?' Catherine asked. She could tell I was a little dejected. 'I don't know, I've not looked at my watch yet, it didn't feel very fast at all,' I said.

I looked down at my Casio Illuminator. I couldn't believe what I saw . . .

19:17

It was over a minute faster than my PB. Wow! Could this really have been down to some simple adjustments to my breathing?

I didn't even know if I was doing it right. I'd not done anything dramatic like switch to nasal breathing, I was still using my mouth. All I'd done was try to control the speed of my breathing and to breathe a little deeper. Yet I'd knocked a whole minute off.

My obsession for wanting to know more about breathing and how to train it was born. I kept asking myself the following:

- Did something as simple as breathing really make that much difference?
- Does the simple act of breathing have that much potential influence on running?
- How much faster could I go if I really invested time and energy in training my breathing?

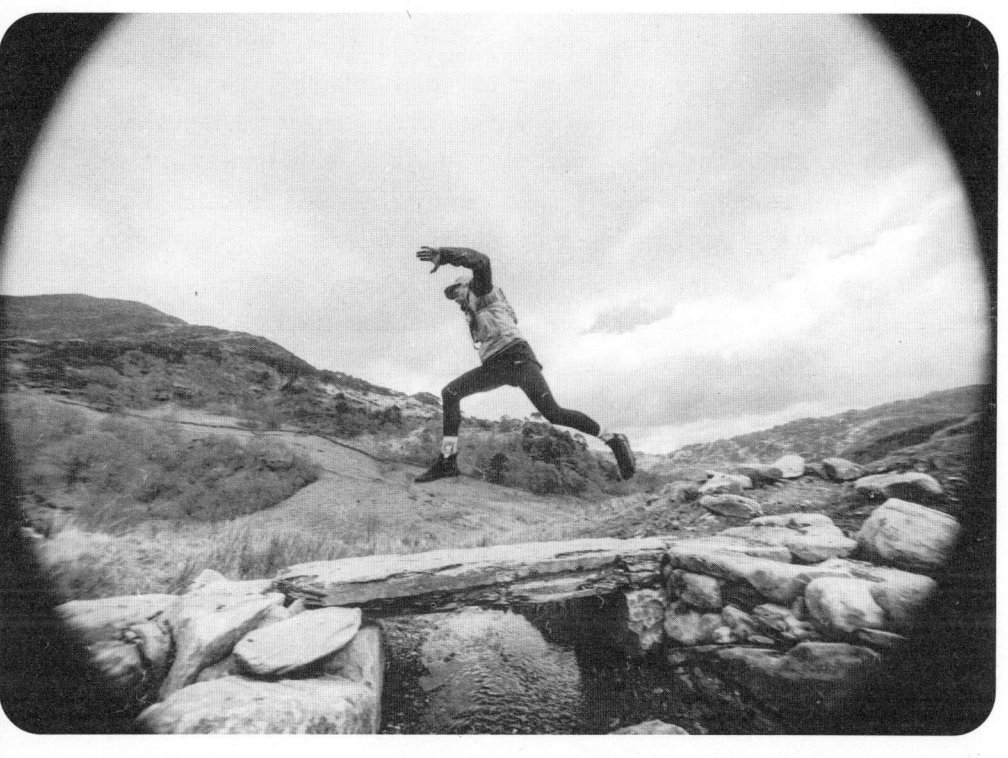

Introduction

That parkrun gave me a little taste, but I wanted more – if just this little bit of breath control helped my running that much, what else can it do? I didn't even know if I was doing it right! I wanted to know how to breathe correctly: what does breathing correctly feel like? How do you know if you are doing it right? I had more and more questions, but no answers.

I started exploring, researching and uncovering the unexpected benefits of optimising breathing by understanding the functional anatomy of the respiratory system. I started training the elements that are adaptable and working out what's most important for improving athletic performance and recovery, both physically and mentally.

I began studying elite runners to discover what they do more naturally than us and why they call breathing their 'superpower'. What do Eliud Kipchoge and David Rudisha have in common? Picture them in your mind, gliding almost effortlessly towards the finish line. Yes, they both hold unbelievable world records for the marathon and 800m, respectively, but what do they have in common? It's not just that they are world record holders; they are totally at ease and in control of their breathing. It looks effortless.

Compare that with someone who finds running hard – they also find breathing very hard. Picture someone struggling at the end of a run, mouth wide open, panting, and they can't control the rate and volume of their breath. It looks the opposite of effortless. It looks so hard that they should probably stop running.

Being in control of your breathing isn't just for the elites like Kipchoge and Rudisha, it's for all of us runners. It's just that we've never been taught how to control our breathing, and no one has ever broken down the process of improving our efficiency and how to use breathing to our advantage rather than being a hinderance.

What does being a 'strong runner' mean to you? It might mean performance improvements and setting PBs. Or it might be more about health and longevity. What you're about to learn is how breathing can play a role in both.

If you're a little sceptical at the start, as I was, be reassured that it's normal to have some doubts that this simple thing called breathing – which happens automatically – could have such an effect. Even Olympic athletes like 400m runner Iwan Thomas expressed a similar sentiment to me: 'I took breathing for granted,' he explained. 'I probably should have been working on my breathing, maybe I was deep breathing when I was listening to my music pre-race, but I just don't know.' Iwan explained that he'd missed out on the latest sports science when he was competing as it just wasn't at the level it is now.

In the opening chapters, we'll look at why breath training has been overlooked in the sports performance world for too long, particularly in Western society, despite breathing being a central pillar to eastern practices like yoga and Qigong. We'll understand why athletes are seeking specialist training from a breathing coach like me, as it's not yet part of a traditional training plan in most sports, especially running.

In this book, we'll unveil the breathing strategies and expose the hidden secrets of breathing the elite athletes are using to gain an edge for their performance. I'll share what I've learned from working with international athletes and teams to improve their physical and mental performance and recovery. In my quest to uncover the breathing strategies that are transforming runners, I've interviewed some of the top and most influential researchers in this field and some of the best runners and coaches to bring you the latest findings and, importantly, what the top athletes are using practically.

Once we have a better understanding of why breathing has been overlooked in the sports performance world, we'll discover what the latest scientific research identifies as most important and trainable for runners.

After learning how to assess your breathing, we outline key breathing techniques and strategies for you to learn and practise to transform your running.

We look at two distinct key opportunities: what is beneficial and optimal **during running**, and breathing protocols to **integrate into your training** for long-term adaptation.

When running, we consider how efficiently you're ventilating, how much oxygen you extract with each breath, breathing mechanics and ribcage position, as well as the effect this has on running posture and force transfer and, ultimately, improved running economy.

For breathing protocols to integrate into your training, we consider long-term adaptation, which ultimately reduces your perception of fatigue and effort, by improving breathing efficiency, lactate tolerance and clearance. For recovery we can enhance reoxygenation of muscle tissues within sessions, as well as nervous system regulation post training.

Your breathing mechanics will even affect spine and hip mobility, relieving pain that you've been putting up with for far too long. Breathing has a rhythm that, when synchronised with your steps, can change your perception of effort, provide free energy and hypnotise you into flow state, also known as being 'in the zone'. Where you're fully immersed in the moment, you're not thinking, everything just happens; it's a magical place of relaxation where our best running performances can be found.

Understanding the why and how of breath training means it's then just a simple case of integrating it into whatever race, event, training session, warm-up or cool down you are doing. The beauty of breathing is that you're always doing it, so there is always an opportunity to adapt your breathing technique to the given situation. This is why the key term I like to use is 'integration'. Frequently, when speaking to runners about breathing, I'm often initially confronted with 'it's not another extra thing I've got to do is it?' The simple answer is no. It's not the case that you have to do a load of extra breath training to get the benefits. You're already breathing in every event or training run you do. We just need to integrate it. When we integrate effectively, we can optimise any training session or run.

A key muscle that's central to our story of breathing, that is misunderstood at best and overlooked at worse, is the diaphragm.

It's the primary muscle of inhalation, who's so important he/she has their own chapter dedicated to them. You're going to learn who your diaphragm is, where he or she lives inside of you and become the best of friends. Your diaphragm is like some sort of superhero you've heard rumours about but just don't know how to call on its power when you need it most – which should be every breath you take.

The benefits you're about to discover go far beyond improving performance and recovery. It's not just about the physical benefits; breathing is linked to your emotional and cognitive state, and it can help calm a racing mind, help you stay focused and control pre-race nerves.

You'll learn 'hacks' that will become secret weapons in races against your opponents, as well as new challenges in training to transform you into a stronger runner. Every coach I've spoken to along the way has said that 'staying relaxed' is the most important thing to become a stronger runner. Guess what opens the door to relaxation? Your breath.

When you're breathing smarter, you stay more relaxed and fluid, which transforms your running. And, importantly, there's the change in mindset. You'll start to realise that you're far more capable than you allow yourself to believe, through the power of this 'untapped mine' that's been hiding inside of you all along: your own breath.

> Jacko is a fantastic coach, who's been part of my coaching team that supported me to multiple gold medals and world records. Learning to breathe better is a game changer for your running.
>
> **Richard Whitehead MBE, paralympic champion and world record holder**

My story – Brain injury to breathing

If you've never thought about breathing, you're not alone – I was just like you. During my 13 years as a professional rugby player in the Championship with Nottingham Rugby, my boyhood team, I never once considered how breathing might be impacting my performance, recovery and mental state. During our hardest pre-season fitness training, where we'd have that horrible metallic taste in the mouth, teeth aching from the extreme anaerobic nature of the brutal conditioning sessions (I did love the challenge of those type of sessions though, as much as they hurt), with our lungs screaming for more air and oxygen, we would have bitten your arm off if you could have taught us how to get more air and oxygen in efficiently by training our breathing. But it just wasn't something that was coached. It wasn't something that was understood. It was overlooked by us all.

My journey into researching, unpicking and trying to understand how breathing affects all aspects of our physiology started once my rugby career had come to an end.

At the start of my 13th season as a professional rugby player in August 2013, I woke up in the hospital waiting area and remember looking at my bright yellow rugby boots, looking to my right, seeing our physio and wondering why was he here with me, thinking *why have I got my boots on in hospital?* With an all-too-familiar sense of feeling disorientated, confused and not knowing why I was in hospital, I said to Michael, our physio, 'I've been knocked out haven't I?' 'Yes,' he replied impatiently.

'I've asked you that question a lot, haven't I?'

'Yes, Jacko, you have!'

This had happened a number of times in my career, but this time it was different. It seemed I suffered a seizure on the training field. A seizure is when you have a 'fit' where, as the neurologist explained, the brain is doing a reset, 'like hitting control, alt, delete on a computer'. This is a common occurrence, apparently, for traumatic brain injuries when there's been a bleed on the brain. I had a small bleed on the brain, but luckily no operation was required. Four months after the injury, the MRI scan revealed it had left a scar on my brain, signalling the end of my rugby career.

Luckily, I don't remember having the seizure, I'd actually lost around two weeks of memory that's never come back. My teammates said it happened on the training field during a game of touch. It was an accident as two of us collided trying to catch the same pass. I'm told it was almost funny initially, but I hit the deck like a sack of potatoes and starting fitting. Everyone was shocked, but luckily, my teammate Shawsy remembered how to put someone in the recovery position and stopped me from swallowing my tongue, while others called the physio over.

I'd been knocked out over 10 times in my rugby career and taken to hospital a number of times, but never had a seizure before. My initial thoughts were about getting back to playing just like I'd always done. I even asked the physio whether I'd be able to play that week!

This time doctors didn't even keep me in hospital overnight, as they did with the previous concussion I'd sustained. I was told to rest up at home but needed 24-hour observation by friends or family, as in the first 24 hours after a brain injury like this, you have a high chance of clotting, which can be life-threatening.

The next 24 hours made it clear this wasn't like any of my other concussions. I remember going to the shop with my sister, who was looking after me, and breaking down in tears because the cognitive demand of choosing what flavour yogurt I wanted was too much for my injured brain. Standing looking at the yogurts, crying my eyes out, I knew it was wrong. I knew I shouldn't be upset by this, but I wasn't in control of my emotions.

There are many symptoms associated with brain injuries. For weeks and months I suffered from fatigue, depression, concentration issues, headaches, sensitivity to lights, cognitive dysfunction and I couldn't tolerate any form of exercise. After the first few weeks I still wasn't getting any better: I remember my wife taking me back to hospital. I was like a zombie, couldn't function in daily life. We'd got married one month before the injury, having been together for 10 years, and I wasn't the man she married. The doctors sent me home, saying there was nothing more they could do, and I just needed to continue to rest.

Weeks turned into months, and I started to realise I was scared to play rugby again. I was trying to follow return-to-play protocols, but exercise kicked off my symptoms anytime I started feeling any better. Eventually, the neurologist who identified the small bleed on my brain from the MRI scan advised that I needed to retire from professional rugby, as the next head trauma could be fatal. I was suffering from an accumulation of previous head injuries.

That decision to retire in January 2014 was the starting point of my recovery. It took the pressure off trying to get back to playing rugby, and I finally accepted that I'd sustained a traumatic brain injury. My focus needed to be on brain health and trying to get out of this zombie state and back to some level of functionality in normal life.

At this point I didn't know if I'd be able to live a normal life. I couldn't stay awake long enough during the day to sustain a nine-to-five job. My recovery came with many challenges. One of which was not knowing how long the recovery would take and how much of a recovery I'd be able to make. There is always this dark cloud of potential cognitive problems later on in life, most commonly the early onset of dementia.

Hence the focus on brain health. Catherine and I started researching important things that were in our control, things like nutrition and gut health. It was a team effort because my recovery affected her as much as it did me. As part of our research into gut health, we came across links between the gut and the brain, which eventually led us to the link between breathing, the brain and the nervous system.

The respiratory centres that control your breathing are situated in your brain stem, smack bang in the middle of your brain. During a traumatic brain injury, the violent shaking of the head with the rebounding of the brain inside your skull disrupts the respiratory centres without you realising. You are aware of the injury because of the symptoms such as depression, fatigue, headaches, etc, but you have no idea that your breathing has been affected. Research shows that your natural breathing rate increases and your breathing becomes shallower without you realising (as reported in the *British Journal of Anaesthesia* in 1968[1]). As a result, your nervous system becomes dysregulated, all of which leads to a reduction in blood flow to the brain and less vital oxygen being delivered, which is essential for recovery and healing.

Re-training my breathing became an important part of my brain health and an essential part of my recovery to restore vital brain functions. Those 6 to 12 months were the most difficult time of my life, and I still don't know if there will be any long-term consequences. However, I am eternally grateful for the traumatic brain injury because what I learned about breathing as a result has helped me get to where I am today.

As you can imagine, that wasn't how I first viewed the injury, as the recovery wasn't straightforward. In fact, it took a few years from the injury in 2013 to stumble upon the importance of breathing. I was sceptical at first – like most people – with the idea that something as simple as breathing could help heal my brain and regulate my nervous system, but I trusted the science I was reading in the research, and I had nothing to lose. I hadn't been given a single piece of advice from any doctors or specialists other than to rest.

Part of my recovery was being able to get back to tolerating exercise, especially running, after 12 months. I'll never forget the first time running since the brain injury without getting headaches – running up to a lookout point at the Fox glacier in New Zealand, while on holiday. Catherine and I were both equally shocked and excited, as we'd had to run to get there before access to the lookout point closed.

The excitement of being able to run again soon slipped into depression, as I was so unfit and not in my best running condition. I was out of breath and couldn't keep up with Catherine whenever we tried to run together. My poor breathing had slipped under the radar, but the demands of running were exposing it. Running became the gateway to training and improving my breathing. As time went on, as I researched further and experimented on myself, my breathing started to transform my running. I went from not being able to run 2km to running ultra-marathons over 200km!

It took some time, years in fact, to go through that recovery process, the earliest part being the hardest. Despite going through some of the darkest times during my recovery, the injury that ended one career ignited another – my brain injury opened my eyes to breathing and the power it has to transform you as a runner.

Without my brain injury, I wouldn't have considered training breathing. I would never have researched it and certainly wouldn't be doing the work I do today. Despite it being the most difficult period in our lives for me and my wife, I thank my brain injury for where it has led me.

> Trail runs, half marathons, long runs – today, I do them all with nasal breathing and a strong, steady breath. But that wasn't always the case. I struggled with asthma for 15 years. Running often felt like a battle against my own lungs, especially in spring when everything bloomed but my breathing shut down.
>
> Everything changed when I learned how to train my breath and return to natural, functional breathing. Through breathwork, I built CO_2 tolerance, calmed my nervous system and discovered a whole new connection to my body. I only wish I had known this when I was younger.
>
> Now, I recover faster, sleep deeper and move with ease and awareness. I feel more resilient – on the trail and in daily life. Breath training didn't just improve my running. It gave me back freedom, confidence and a whole new level of joy in movement.
>
> **Jennyfer Haas, runner and breathing coach**

CHAPTER 1

What is breathing?

Breathing is automatic. We don't need to think about it; it just happens. It's so vital to life that it needs to be autonomic (happen automatically); so it still happens when we are doing all the other stuff life demands of us.

I watched my father take his last breath at home; it was a deeply sad and powerful moment. It was a hammer blow to the heart at the same time as magnifying the life-giving power of our breathing which we otherwise take for granted.

Describing breathing as 'simple' doesn't do this life-giving multistage process the credit it deserves. Breathing has the power to keep you calm and make you feel relaxed; it has influence over your nervous system to make you feel more stressed; it affects your brain states and cognition, your blood pressure, blood flow, how your heart is beating and the vital oxygen delivery needed when running. As an underlying autonomic process within the body, it influences so many bodily systems and our overall physiology – it's far from simple.

That said, we can explain the act of breathing in a nutshell. Breathing, or ventilation, is simply defined as the act of moving air into and out of the lungs – that's it. The end.

But if that was it, then this would be a very short book. How the air moves in and out of the lungs, the volume and speed of it, how it reaches the airways, the order and way in which the lungs fill up are all part of the magic of breathing.

The most common focus of breathing is the vital gas exchange that occurs with each breath. Oxygen (O_2) comes in and carbon dioxide (CO_2)

goes out – that is the overly simplified version our science teachers tell us (I know, I was a secondary school science teacher for one year!). But about 75% of the oxygen you breathe in, you immediately breathe out with your next exhale, depending on how efficient your breathing is. If you are more efficient, you can extract more oxygen from the lungs per breath, but more on that later.

Each breath has an inhale and an exhale as part of its cycle. The purpose of the inhale is to bring air into the lungs, of which 20.9% is oxygen, which is vital for life and energy. The oxygen travels through your airway, down your windpipe into the lungs, where the bronchi branch off to either the left or right lung, passing through smaller and smaller pipes (bronchioles) to the tiny air sacs (alveoli), where the oxygen passes, via diffusion, into the blood. The blood then carries the oxygen to all the cells of your body.

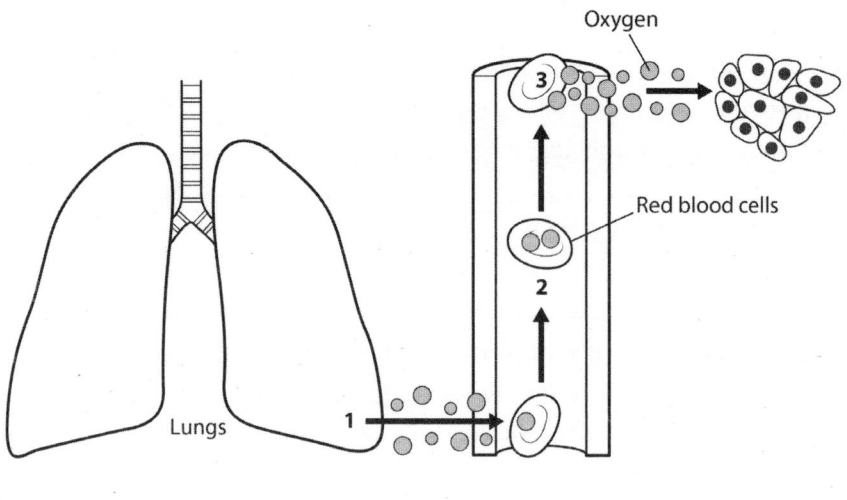

1 From the lungs into the blood
2 Carried in the bloodstream
3 Delivered to the cells

Oxygen passing from the lungs is diffused into the lungs and transported to the cells

In simple terms, air enters the lungs with each inhale via a change in internal pressure relative to the external air pressure. When we increase the volume inside of us during an inhalation, we decrease pressure and air moves from high pressure to low pressure.

So, during an inhalation, the increase in volume in your chest cavity (thorax) decreases the pressure relative to atmospheric pressure (air outside the body), thereby drawing air in.

How we expand the chest cavity to draw air in affects the efficiency of our breathing and oxygen uptake from the lungs. During the inhale, the diaphragm – which plays a key role in the story of breathing and is nestled below the chest cavity at the bottom of the ribcage – is supposed to move down and out as it contracts, drawing air into the lungs.

When we exhale, ideally the diaphragm relaxes and moves back up. Our chest cavity reduces in size, and air is forced out, removing carbon dioxide from the lungs, which our body has created, as we exhale.

At rest our exhalation is relatively passive, relying on the natural elasticity of the lungs, ribcage and diaphragm; yet during exercise such as running, exhalation becomes active. There is increased movement of the ribs downwards and inwards, requiring activation from expiratory muscles, including the internal intercostal and oblique muscles.

During exercise both the demand for oxygen and the production of carbon dioxide from cellular respiration (energy production) increase. The dynamics of how you take each breath affect the efficiency of it. The less efficiently you breathe, the more air you have to ventilate.

The way the lungs are structured means there is a much greater proportion and density of those important tiny air sacs (alveoli), where the oxygen needs to get to, towards the bottom of the lungs. This is an important point to understand when it comes to the efficiency of breathing.

The shape of the branching airways in our lungs are like the branches of a tree – if the tree was upside down. Like how a tree has more leaves at the end of all the branches, our lungs have more alveoli at the end of the bronchioles. Interestingly, the gas exchange is the opposite way round. With trees, the leaves take in carbon dioxide and release oxygen, whereas in our lungs, the alveoli take in oxygen and release carbon dioxide.

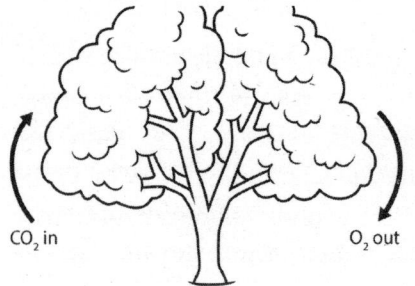 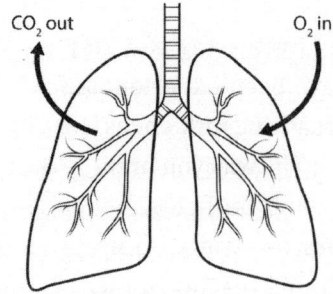

Our lungs are structured like an upside-down tree, with the opposite exchange of O_2 and CO_2

Breathing, however, isn't just about the vital oxygen necessary for life. When running, breathing does indeed enable the delivery of oxygen, but its power to transform your running performance goes way beyond its delivery of oxygen.

Overly simplifying breathing has restricted our exploration of its use in sports performance. When we overly simplify even the simplest of things, like breathing, we miss out on important nuances. With breathing, I've seen how these nuances can transform an athlete's physical and mental capacity.

Our breathing is interwoven within our nervous system. It's in constant communication with it and our body. Think about it: when you are stressed, how do you feel? You feel tense. How do you breathe? Your breathing is fast and shallow. How do you run when you feel stressed? You're tense, lethargic and frustrated.

Our breathing affects how we think, how we feel and how we perform. For example, if I'm breathing inefficiently and therefore have to breathe much faster, not only do I find talking to my friend as we run difficult because I feel out of breath, I've also got an increased heart rate. Faster breathing leads to an increased 'fight or flight' stress response and a faster heart rate. This increase in stress response increases muscle tone, so you feel tense and tight, rather than relaxed and fluid. You'll feel tired and fatigue sooner. It will be harder to stay focused and concentrate because your whole system is working harder. The longing for flow state will be but a fleeting thought, as all you can think about is *when will this run be over?*

Even once the run is over, the increased stress response you'll have been experiencing will also affect your ability to recover, as your breathing influences the state of your nervous system.

The way you breathe even affects how much vital stability you create around your core and pelvis. This can transform tight, painful hips and improve your running economy, as your ability to transfer important ground reaction forces becomes more efficient, propelling you forwards effortlessly and, ironically, using less oxygen.

Put simply, yes, your breathing is automatic, but you can also take conscious control of it to improve your 'auto setting'. If you are just letting your auto setting take over, you're missing out on the ability to control and change all those key factors that breathing can influence.

BREATHING RATE FACTS

Ever noticed or wondered why you feel more out of breath when you go on a run while you feel stressed? Both increase breathing rate...

Breathing rate is so important that researchers now suggest it's a better marker for rate of perceived exertion (RPE) than heart rate measured by expensive watches or even lactate levels that need to be measured in a laboratory![1]

Here's how breathing rate changes, on average, from resting to walking to running.[2]

- At rest = 14bpm (breaths per minute)
- Walking speed 6km/hr = 20bpm
- Running speed 12km/hr = 35bpm

These numbers are based on 'normal' value but are not necessarily optimal.

Some of us are breathing as if we're jogging, even when we are simply at rest. That's not a good starting place for your breathing! Emerging evidence is highlighting the importance of controlling breathing rate during running. A 2023 study stated, 'respiratory frequency reflects physical effort and is sensitive to changes in exercise tolerance' and, interestingly, 'it has a rate of increase during exercise that is negatively associated with exercise tolerance'.[3] Meaning the faster you breathe while running, the harder it feels, and you'll be less resilient to the demands of exercise.

When you are more stressed, you'll breathe faster. When you are less efficient at breathing, you'll breathe faster. The faster you breathe, the more fatigued you feel, the more out of breath you feel and the harder it is to relax when running.

Are you in control of your breathing, or is your breathing controlling you?

Working with Jacko truly opened my eyes to the power of breathing in our lives. It's not just about breathing to survive – it's about being fully aware of how each breath impacts our body and mind throughout the day.

With his guidance, I realised that by simply learning to breathe more efficiently, I could significantly improve my performance, both physically and mentally.

Jacko is incredibly passionate about what he does. He teaches with purpose and genuine care, helping you grow step by step – from simple breathing techniques to more advanced practices, always tailored to where you are on your journey. I'm deeply grateful to have crossed paths with him. His knowledge, dedication, and passion for helping others truly make a difference.

Santi Carreras, Argentina international (Rugby Union)

CHAPTER 2

Smarter breathing

When you learn to breathe smarter, you discover the many benefits breathing can have on your running, whatever your goal. Whenever you're running, you're breathing, and when you know how to optimise your breathing, you transform your running.

Rudisha breathed differently

Anyone who watched David Rudisha smash the 800m world record at the London 2012 Olympics witnessed something so surprising that we all missed it.

He was so composed from start to finish, fluid and effortless in stride. Never straining, almost looking like he could have tried a little harder. A true mark of class. The type of performance you'd expect from an all-time great.

Even as he crossed the finish line, smashing the 800m world record, he didn't look at all out of breath. In fact, he never looked out of breath at any point in the race. As they came around the final bend, everyone else behind him lost control of their breathing and, subsequently, their running form, mouths wide open, strain on their faces and bodies rocking from side to side. But not Rudisha. Rudisha was different.

You never saw him lose control of his breathing, whereas everyone behind him seemed to 'blow a gasket'. As their panting increased with their mouths getting wider, so too did the gap to Rudisha.

We couldn't fail to notice Rudisha's unforgettable performance, but we didn't notice that he was breathing differently to everyone else in the race. I remember watching the race, and I couldn't believe that the guy who had just set the world record wasn't even out of breath as he crossed the finish line. I even said to my wife, 'Catherine, what doping is this guy doing? Look, he's not even out of breath, he could at least pretend, it's a joke!'

I, like many still do now, equated being completely out of breath – heavy mouth panting – as a sign that you'd emptied the tank and given it everything you had. If that was true, then David Rudisha just took it easy and smashed the world record. Imagine if he'd actually tried hard, how much faster could he have gone? I laugh now at my own ignorance in thinking *why doesn't the 800m world record holder breathe like I do at the end of my 20-minute parkrun.* Maybe not getting completely out of breath is a key to staying relaxed for good running performance?

I'm sure you're all aware Rudisha was giving it his all – it was the fastest 800m in history after all – but how come he wasn't out of breath? Everyone else in the race was, what was he doing differently? Watching the race 12 years later and looking specifically at his breathing compared with everyone else in the race, it was very clear. So clear and obvious now, I can't believe we missed it at the time. He hardly ever opened his mouth. But back in 2012, I'd not yet had the traumatic brain injury that ended my rugby career, so I'd not started my discovery of the impact and power of breathing.

Now I'm not suggesting that simply keeping his mouth shut was the reason Rudisha set that world record, but what I am suggesting is that we observed one person doing something different with their breathing who was head and shoulders above everyone else.

Breathing can be trained

After my professional rugby career ended abruptly from my brain injury and I'd recovered enough to start a new career, I retrained as a strength and conditioning coach, working with elite and international athletes and teams. It helped me develop a unique perspective regarding breathing; rather than just dismissing it due to its autonomic nature, I look for the opportunities to train and optimise it like any other system in the body. That, however, hasn't always been the case, and I, like many people, generally overlooked breathing in my coaching for years.

One of those elite runners I supported as a strength and conditioning coach is the reason I first met marathon expert and running coach Dr Martin Yelling years ago. Dr Yelling has been in the game a long time and has a wealth of experience coaching runners of all abilities. I wanted to pick his brain specifically about breathing for runners. 'You only think about breathing when it's a problem,' he explained. He continued: 'When you are gassing out and sucking in air from every and any hole, you'd love to know how to do it better. But I've been running marathons and coaching marathon runners for 40 years and never once has someone explained to me and showed me how I can improve my breathing.'

Considering your breathing muscles take up around 15% or more of your total oxygen consumption during running, and knowing what I now know about breathing smarter, it's crazy we don't devote time to training it. The more intensely you run, the more oxygen your muscles need, including your breathing muscles. If you're breathing inefficiently, you'll need more oxygen and your breathing muscles will have to work harder. Not only that, if those breathing muscles start to fatigue, they require more oxygen and 'steal' blood that should be going to your legs for running due to an autonomic reflex called the metaboreflex.[1] Yet, often we don't even consider it, let alone actually train our breathing muscles. Until now!

By the end of our interview Dr Yelling expressed this sentiment with me: 'Breathing is the most fundamental thing we have to do, and when we are running you are only going to do more of it, it's crazy we've never considered training it.' Despite my initial scepticism I totally agree. Don't you?

At school we learn the importance of oxygen; it's vital to life and every cell in your body. Oxygen is so important that breathing is an automatic process. So we don't think about it, which lulls us into overlooking the potential to train and optimise it. Yet the beauty of breathing and the respiratory system is that yes, it is part of the autonomic nervous system

(ANS) and happens automatically, but it's also within our conscious control. We can choose to take control of our breathing and, by doing so, take control of our nervous system's response to running. The very fact that we can control our breathing means we can choose to change it. If we can change it, we can train it. If we can train it, we can improve it. We can make it more efficient; we can use it to our advantage. We can optimise it to transform our running.

Yet, we take it for granted and allow the 'auto' function to run riot when we strap on our running trainers. As James Earls, author of *Born to Walk*, explains, other animals don't have quite the same control over their breathing like we do. I first met James and heard him speak on the evolution of respiratory physiology at a conference in 2022 where we were both presenting. He explained how a four-legged animal, such as a dog, has to breathe in sync with its running (locomotion) – inhaling when the legs extend and exhaling as the legs come together, compressing the ribcage to expel the air. They don't have the luxury of controlling the mechanics of their breathing, the speed of their breathing or anything else we'll uncover in later chapters. We do – but we're not taking advantage of it.

When considering that we can train our breathing to improve our running, it makes sense to look at what elite runners, such as David Rudisha, do differently to us amateur runners, if anything.

The elite athlete's best-kept secret

One thing that stood out when studying runners' breathing is that there's a significant difference been elite and amateurs. When you zoom in and look past the seemingly effortless running technique of an elite runner and instead focus on their breathing, you'll notice almost nothing. It just looks easy for them; they certainly aren't struggling like the rest of us when we attempt our first ever parkrun or are striving for a new 10km PB. Yes, they are clearly fitter and better conditioned than us, but what is different about their breathing? Are there certain things they are doing and aware of that we aren't? Why haven't we heard them talking about it? One former Olympic triathlon coach said to me, 'Athletes and coaches are always looking for incremental gains, breathing is one of them, and the elite athletes don't want to share it.' It's a fair point, if it really helps that much you probably aren't going to share that with the world and your competitors. But there is a lot we can learn by simply observing elite runners.

Ever had that feeling you just can't get enough air in when you're trying to beat your PB on a run? If we stop for a moment and think about those elite runners who are calm and effortlessly in control of their breathing, they don't appear to be getting more air in than us. In fact, they almost look like they are breathing less air than me! Are they more efficient with the oxygen in their body? How do they do that?

Well, something that is jumping out of the new flurry of research into breathing strategies and respiratory physiology within running is that an elite runner doesn't necessarily ventilate (breathe) a larger volume of air than an amateur runner at a relative pace or intensity. It's the way they ventilate. The way they get the air in is different. It's slower, it's more controlled, and it's more efficient.[2] How they do that mechanically, we'll unpack in the coming chapters.

It's natural for our initial thoughts to focus on how much or how well we can get oxygen into our lungs and through our blood to our muscles. As we'll see, that's a significant part of it, but it's by far from the only way breathing influences our running performance. A recent study from 2023, 'Sports Performance and Breathing Rate: What Is the Connection?', shows that just as breathing can have a limiting effect on performance when performed poorly or inefficiently, it can also help regulate our psychological state when we know how to control it. The study noted that controlling a consistent respiratory rate when exercising helps maintain an 'adequate oxygen supply to the muscles, proper elimination of waste products, regulation of the heart rate, and improved focus and concentration, all of which are essential for achieving peak athletic performance'.[3]

If we are 'bad' at breathing it can limit us, but if we are good at it, breathing can enhance our running performance. Breathing is not just physiological; it also affects our mental state. Interestingly, every running coach I've spoken to when asked, 'What is the most important thing for runners?' all responded with 'being able to stay relaxed', which is both physiological and psychological. Breathing influences both.

If being able to stay relaxed is the most important thing any runner can do to transform their running, then breathing really could become your superpower, as Paralympic champion and world record holder Richard Whitehead explained when I asked him how breathing helps his running. When you can't control your breathing, it's very hard to stay relaxed because of the effect a fast breathing rate has on your ANS (autonomic nervous system) and stress response.

Ultra-runner, coach and author Brian MacKenzie has described breathing as 'the remote control of the nervous system'. We know that faster breathing rates speed up the heart rate, activating the sympathetic nervous system – better known as the 'fight or flight' response. We've all felt and experienced the fight or flight response. It's essentially 'up-regulating', which is certainly not relaxing. When you activate the sympathetic nervous system your muscle tone increases automatically, causing the muscles to contract (particularly in flexion tone, which are muscles on the front side of the body), among other bodily changes. If you want to stay relaxed but aren't aware of your breathing, especially your breathing rate, then you're potentially fighting a losing battle against your ANS. Not only is it harder to relax, the increase in flexion tone causes you to lose your long, tall and efficient running form as you start to shrink. If you are inefficient with your breathing, put very simply, you have to do more of it, which results in more tension. Conversely, if you're smart with your breathing and train it to be more efficient, breathing can be calmer, and you stay more relaxed. Like the elite runners.

Sometimes people argue 'you shouldn't mess with something that's automatic like breathing'. But just because something is automatic doesn't mean it's optimal. Nigel Beach is a physiotherapist working in elite sports in New Zealand and Australia with some of the greatest athletes in the world. In our interview he explained, 'The natural physiological response to running is fast, shallow, mouth breathing as part of the stress response. Your ANS doesn't know if you're running away from a bear or trying to get a personal best in your 5km. All it knows is the "stress response" which isn't optimal breathing when you start to push yourself.'

We've all felt the stress response and how our breathing is affected in that stressed state – it's faster and shallower. When we get to that point where we're totally out of breath, panting and can't control our breathing, it's our body's way of making us stop. The Central Governor Theory, proposed by exercise scientist Professor Tim Noakes, explains the concept of the brain trying to protect the organism. It makes sense if you think about it logically. Your body doesn't want the stress of trying to break your 5km or 10km PB. So, it would be crazy for it to breathe in a way that allows you to stress it further. It wouldn't be a safe automatic response. Another reason why consciously controlling your breathing could benefit exercise and running performance when you are pushing your limits.

An interesting question to ask is 'am I actually any good at breathing?' It's an interesting question because, if like me when I started this journey, you have no idea of what 'good breathing' is and therefore no way to make a reliable assessment, you might just assume that you're ok. I never had any issues with my breathing until my brain injury. Respiratory and sleep scientist Martin McPhilimey explained that one of the reasons breathing has been overlooked from a clinical perspective is because 'if someone is fit and healthy and their breathing falls within normalised data, then it's assumed their breathing is fine'.

But fine isn't necessarily optimal. I don't just want my running technique to be 'fine', I want it to be good, better even, great if possible, and I'll work on it. That applies to my approach to breathing. I don't want to be satisfied with it being fine, I want to know how to breathe optimally. I want to know how the elite do it better, so I can learn from them – and I'm sure you do too.

You'll learn later (*see* chapter 7) how to do a full assessment of your breathing, but for now let me shed some light on why assuming breathing is fine may limit its power to optimise your performance. On a practical level, one of the problems is that our inefficiency when breathing at rest can go completely unnoticed. At rest a typical breathing rate is around 10–18 breaths per minute with around half a litre of air per breath. It's not particularly fast and each breath is pretty small in volume, so we don't notice it much, meaning you don't realise that your breathing is inefficient until you start exercising. By then it's potentially too late to do anything about it, as Dr John Dickinson – sports and exercise science physiologist at the University of Kent, who's worked with Olympic athletes – explains in the book *The Lost Art of Running:* 'good breathing habits at rest will promote good breathing patterns during running . . . Breathing should be as automatic as possible and so entraining these good breathing patterns at rest will help continue them during exercise'.[4]

How breathing smarter helps

The latest research shows we can optimise oxygen efficiency by how we ventilate, highlighting that elite runners do it differently to us. A more efficient, controlled breathing rate also helps regulate the nervous system when running, which can help your physiological state but also your cognitive and mental state, leading to better focus and concentration, while staying relaxed. That's breathing smarter.

Related to relaxation is finding rhythm in our running, which you'll learn through something called Locomotor-Respiratory Coupling (LRC). Your breathing can be the gateway to finding your rhythm, accessing flow state and even save you energy when your steps and breath are in beautiful synchronisation. It's hard to stay relaxed when it feels like you can't get enough air into your lungs. You will learn what is creating that sensation of being out of breath physiologically and how the way you're breathing can change what that sensation feels like. You will also learn how that affects your emotional and psychological state and even your perception of effort.

If your airway is restricted, this will massively impact how air is coming into your body and your lungs. You'll learn about an overlooked muscle that Dr Lomas, a biological dentist, called 'the most important muscle in the human body' because of the effect it has on your airway. I'll teach you how to train it in order to strengthen your airway.

Your diaphragm is going to be a leading actor in our story of breathing smarter to transform your running. When you harness the power of your diaphragm and combine it with controlling the speed of your breathing, you become more efficient. The power of your diaphragm doesn't stop there; it also helps to generate pressure within your trunk that not only helps stabilise your spine and pelvis when running but also enhances force transfer when your foot strikes the floor to propel yourself forward. Using the power of your diaphragm also requires you to optimise your ribcage position, which also helps with running form and posture. Combining all of this ultimately helps to improve your running economy.

Not only will you learn and feel how to activate your diaphragm correctly and use it to make your breathing more efficient (in chapter 8), you'll feel how it can improve mobility in two key areas for runners: your thoracic spine and your hips. Your neck, back or hip pain and tightness might just dissolve as the relationship with your diaphragm blossoms.

It doesn't stop there. Interestingly, the breath can also be used as a training tool. Patrick McKeown, author of *The Oxygen Advantage*, spoke to me about using breathing to 'add a training load'. We can choose to do something specific such as breathe only through our nose during certain training session intensities to create longer-term adaptations. In chapter 4, we'll even explore the benefits of not breathing at all, as we uncover the benefits of integrating breath-holding into particular running sessions. This has been the focus of researcher Xavier Woorons, who worked with Olympic athletes ahead of the Paris Olympics in 2024 to optimise their performance and recovery.

If you're going to add an extra load to some training, it's also important to learn to recover smarter. Breathing has a direct relationship with both heart rate and perceived exertion, and you'll learn in chapter 12 how to use breathing to help improve recovery. We'll explore recovery both in the moment within a training session, such as a rest period between sets of intervals, and to promote enhanced recovery post-session and between training days by down-regulating the nervous system with your breath.

As well as providing you with practical tools and the opportunity to implement them, in the penultimate chapter, I'll give advice and examples of how you can seamlessly integrate them into various training sessions. You are already breathing whenever you're running, so we'll integrate the techniques into what you're already doing – no one wants to have more work to do, and you don't have to. I'll explain practically which techniques are best suited to different training sessions as well as nuances that depend on the type of race and distance of event you are taking part in.

Finally, it's not just about breaking PBs and optimising performance. The way you breathe influences your health (importantly your heart) and your enjoyment of running. Many of us engage in exercise and running because we want to be healthier; we want to live longer and live well for longer. Yet we adopt an unhealthy breathing pattern when we perform the exercise that we're hoping will help us be healthier. It is actually a bit of an oxymoron if you think about it: breathing unhealthily while trying to do something supposed to be healthy. Plus, we'll learn from Professor George Dallam that if your breathing is healthier, you're less likely to pick up respiratory illnesses, get ill and miss training sessions which, in the long term, harvests more consistent training and ultimately progress in performances.

For those interested in health and longevity over performance, it's also about enjoyment, making running feeling easier. In some cases, your poor breathing isn't just stopping you from staying relaxed, it's worse than that. It's actually a barrier to you enjoy running because we feel so out of breath as soon as we start. We brush it off saying 'I'm just unfit' and 'running isn't for me'. Or is it that your breathing is restricting your ability to run? Running is probably one of the most natural forms of exercise you can do – and, for most, you can just go outside and run. But inefficient breathing means it can become a barrier for your running or any type of exercise as soon as you start. Improving the quality and efficiency of your breathing will not only improve your performance and recovery but you'll enjoy your exercise and running more. It feels amazing not to be out of breath when you're running. It's far more enjoyable when you can smile and enjoy the experience of running, instead of panting out of breath.

As runners shouldn't we be good at breathing?

It appears that more and more runners are starting to become aware of needing help with their breathing. Where do we turn to these days when looking for answers? YouTube.

Anna Harding from 'The Running Channel' explained in our interview that during some research for their content creation, one of the questions that people are searching on YouTube is 'how to breathe when running'. Anna explained that it's a question likely asked by more amateur runners or those just starting out, but it certainly doesn't have a clear and concise answer. We discussed that it might also be down to a lack of education, understanding and coaching.

The faster you run, the more challenging your breathing is. If you don't know how to control your breathing effectively when challenged, it won't automatically improve.

So contrary to what you might think, going out for a run and feeling out of breath might not help you improve your breathing as much as you thought. If you are unaware you are breathing badly and you challenge your poor breathing by running, your breathing is only going to get worse with compensatory breathing patterns developing. You will just get better and stronger at suboptimal compensatory breathing.

This was highlighted in a 2023 study that showed 90.6% of the athletic population displayed dysfunctional breathing during biomechanics assessments.[5] Because we aren't taught about correct breathing during exercise (we just assume that because it's automatic, it's fine), we're totally unaware of how to control it during exercise. Therefore, we allow compensatory breathing patterns to take over, which become ingrained, strengthening dysfunctional breathing during running and affecting breathing in our day-to-day lives and at rest. Another study from 2022 noted that 40% of runners have issues with their breathing during running that restricts their performance, 'as a result of cascading physiological phenomena, possibly causing negative psychological states or barriers to participation'.[6]

Unless you're like Ellis Bland, top British fell runner, who knows the importance of breathing for both his ability to stay calm in warm-ups to control pre-race nerves and also manage the intensity of elite fell running. He explained two key things to me: 'breathing deeper with the diaphragm when it's needed' and the importance of avoiding shallow breathing. But unlike most runners I've met and interviewed, Ellis has a slightly unfair advantage. His partner is an international yoga teacher, helping people all over the world to breathe better. He understands how to mechanically ventilate efficiently; he understands the importance of breathing for his performance; and he's one of the best fell runners in the United Kingdom. We aren't all as lucky as Ellis to have a yoga teacher by our side.

However, you do now have the advice from this book, some of which will help you in the immediate term, while other strategies are for integrating into your training in the long term. A common example of seeing an immediate improvement is Tess Elias, an elite trail runner who came second at the world-renowned Ultra-Trail Snowdonia (UTS) 100km in 2024, qualifying for the prestigious UTMB around Mont Blanc. Tess, despite being a phenomenal ultra-runner, suffers with asthma, which was apparent the first time we tried working on her breathing. Runners who have trouble with breathing or have never worked on it, rather than using their diaphragm as Ellis Bland described, are typically upper chest dominant, especially when breathing is fast, rather than relaxed and controlled. After some work on her airway, tongue position and breathing mechanics, her breathing was transformed by activating her diaphragm for 5–10 minutes. On a short hill run we retested her breathing. She was more in control and looked and felt much more relaxed. Oxygen was getting to her legs more effectively (measured with near-infrared spectrometry device), and she recovered much faster as heart rate reduced to 79bpm after two minutes compared with 102bpm the first time we did the run.

A huge improvement in recovery and more oxygen reaching her muscles when she optimised her breathing dynamics in real time. This was a short-term intervention; the real magic happens when, over time, longer-term training adaptation occurs.

What if you trained your breathing as well as your running?

It's likely you've never actually trained your breathing. You've become fitter, faster and a better runner up to this point, but we're leaving money on the table if we don't train our breathing like we train our running. Don't fall into the trap of assuming that because you've been running and training hard, it's automatically making you better at breathing. Research suggests it's actually more likely you've developed less efficient breathing mechanics and you're not using the power of the diaphragm to its fullest potential.[7]

What could you achieve with your running if you weren't always running out of breath? The next step on this journey of using breathing to transform your running is a shift in mindset. I get it. I was the most sceptical at the start. How can something as simple as breathing, which happens automatically, transform my running? If training your breathing was so helpful, wouldn't we have heard more about it by now? Wouldn't there be loads of research to prove it? Well yes, there is, and that is exactly where we are going in the next chapter, looking at why breathing has been overlooked and what has caused the researchers to make a recent U-turn. It comes with a little warning though: it might challenge your current way of thinking, and so I want you to take a calm nasal breath and approach the next chapter with an open mind.

Key takeaways

- Don't assume training hard and breathing hard makes you better at breathing.
- As breathing affects your nervous system, it not only impacts your physical performance and physiology but also your mental performance and psychology.
- Elite runners breathe more efficiently, and we can learn from them and train our breathing to be more efficient.
- Relaxation is key to better running, and breathing is a direct link to relaxation.

Since working with Jacko the impact he's had on my mental and physical feeling has been transformational. The techniques and education he has taught me has opened my eyes into how to breathe properly in certain positions and situations to improve my performance.

Whether that's mobility, controlling my breathing in the heat of the game or down-regulation breathing, the impact has been absolutely brilliant. I can't thank him enough for his help.

George Ford, England Rugby

CHAPTER 3

Why breathing has been overlooked, and why it's not your fault

Elite runners don't just run better than us, they breathe better than us. They are able to ventilate more efficiently and deliver more oxygen with less effort. Yet the science and research has long overlooked breathing because we've made assumptions about this automatic process. Now we're seeing some scientists make a U-turn and you're about to find out why.

Breathing differently

It's clear that elite runners and athletes around the world are doing different things with their breathing that we're not. It's been going on longer than you might expect, for example, why was one of the greatest distance runners of all time, Emil Zátopek, the 'Czech Locomotive', who set 18 world records in the 1940s and 1950s, holding his breath and running as far as he could in his training? Was there something about taking control of certain aspects of his breathing that created favourable adaptations for performance? Did he realise something others had missed? After all, he was the first person in history to break the 29-minute mark for 10,000m over 70 years ago!

That is just one (fairly extreme) example we'll unpick in later chapters. There are plenty more ways we can use our breathing to help improve performance, maintain relaxation, reduce fatigue, feel less out of breath and recover faster, to name a few. But first I'd like us to go on a little journey to find out why breathing has been overlooked and why some of us are still dismissive of it.

Why has breathing been overlooked?

I've always asked the same question to every expert I've met and interviewed along the journey, 'Why has breathing been overlooked?' There doesn't appear to be any single reason. Along with a lack of research, one reason is the misconception or assumption that how you're breathing during exercise doesn't make a difference to things such as oxygen extraction in the lungs and delivery to the muscles. Respiratory and sleep clinical scientist Martin McPhilimey agrees the research has overlooked breathing because it's not 'popular'. He believes that there is 'an assumption that if someone is fit then their breathing is "ideal", yet there are a large number of athletes that struggle.'

Assumptions often lead us down the wrong path, and I could sense some frustration from Martin that these assumptions within the science world were holding it back from better understanding the impact of breathing on athletic performance. The tide is starting to turn, however; a review paper in December 2023 highlighted that breathing has been overlooked: 'the importance of breathing monitoring is currently underappreciated in the field of sport and exercise, partially because the pulmonary system has long been considered overbuilt for exercise'.[1] Yet research into breathing can be difficult because it's not easy to measure and requires a whole-body approach. Author of *Born to Walk* James Earls explained: 'the whole body is involved, pressure in different cavities for example, it can't be done at present so there's a lack of research, meaning there's a lack of exploring . . . my frustration is so few people in research have a systems approach.'

Further frustration from James Earls that matched Martin McPhilimey and my own. I'm starting to get a sense from the world of research that one of our biggest challenges is the closed mindsets we develop when assumptions become accepted and morph into a 'truth', blinding us from seeing the full picture. Researching breathing has its challenges, but science should be questioning our thinking rather than agreeing with assumptions. If we're wrong, we have to be prepared to put our hand up and say, 'We got it wrong; breathing is more important than we thought.'

Minimal effort principle

The minimal effort principle could be one of those assumptions holding us back from untapping the potential of our respiratory system and how we ventilate. The principle asserts that autonomic control of our breathing during exercise limits tidal volume (size of each breath) to around 50–60% of our vital capacity (maximal volume of one breath at rest), and instead increases respiratory rate, as the metabolic cost of a large tidal volume is greater than the inefficiency caused by an increased respiratory rate.[2] This particularly comes into play during our second ventilatory threshold during VO_2 max testing (an incremental exercise test to determine the maximum amount of oxygen utilised in one minute) where breathing demand increases disproportionally as intensity and pace ramp up and, typically, we see an increase in breathing rate rather than tidal volume (size of breath).

The minimal effort principle has one potential problem – what your body is able to do most efficiently is based on what it finds easiest (least effort) out of the options available. Take breathing mechanics for example: what if you've developed really strong accessory breathing muscles but your diaphragm is relatively weak in comparison? Or your ribcage is tight, with ribs stuck and your diaphragm all 'jacked up' and restricted. Which will your brain choose to fire when working on the minimal effort principle? The depth of your breath and ability to efficiently increase tidal volume will surely be dependent on the efficiency of your breathing mechanics, the strength, function and endurance of your diaphragm (and other respiratory muscles), as well as the mobility of your ribcage to expand.

Air follows the path of least resistance, and the brain will choose the accessory breathing muscles to hike the ribcage up and increase breathing rate, rather than increase tidal volume by drawing air deeper into the lower portion of the lungs with the diaphragm, if the diaphragm itself is restricted. It becomes familiar for the brain, a path well-trodden, so to speak. The brain likes what's easy and familiar. The minimal effort principle assumes your body will select the most efficient way for you to ventilate, but it can only choose from what you have available, not necessarily from what's optimal.

So what is it that elite runners are doing that is optimal and more efficient? The latest research shows that elite athletes can continue to increase tidal volume all the way up to exhaustion in a VO_2 max test.[3] Typically, tidal volume peaks at around 50–60% of vital capacity (maximal breath volume at rest), but can be as low as 35% in untrained people because when working to exhaustion, they instead just breathe faster and faster.[4,5] Yet elite athletes can increase the size of their breath (tidal volume) to as much as 70% of vital capacity.[6] It's clear elite runners take a different approach to ventilating as demand increases. Their minimal effort comes from increasing tidal volume rather than simply increasing the speed of breathing, which is what restricts an amateur runner's ability to ventilate efficiently and stay relaxed.

If you learned to be more efficient with your breathing like an elite runner and had that as an option, wouldn't your minimal effort automatic choice be different for you too?

It's important to point out this is only one aspect of how breathing can affect your running. It's only looking at the acute oxygen extraction at the lungs and delivery to your muscles while running. It has the most scepticism around it, hence why I want to address it early on. The efficiency of oxygen delivery is affected by speed of breathing, which also has an effect on other aspects of our physiology and psychology when running. That all-important ability to maintain relaxation is harder the faster you're breathing. So although it's just one aspect, it has knock-on effects to other benefits through control of the breathing rate.

Overbuilt or overlooked?

I love the quote by scientist and philosopher Carlo Rovelli, 'What's important is not to be right, it's to try to understand', because it highlights the need for an open mindset in science, to be curious to possibilities.[7] Norman Doidge, author of *The Brain That Changes Itself*, wrote about Dr Paul Bach-y-Rita who was ridiculed in the 1980s for suggesting that the brain can make new neural pathways. He was the first to suggest the theory of neuroplasticity after helping his father recover from a debilitating stroke, and he got laughed out of the medical world. Yet now everyone is like *oh yeah, neuroplasticity, yeah, of course mate, the brain can change, of course*. It's now widely accepted, but it wasn't always the case – just ask Dr Paul Bach-y-Rita.

A similar story of breathing stems from 1985 when Professor Dempsey delivered a lecture to colleagues titled 'Is the lung built for exercise?' He was a pioneer, challenging the status quo and current thinking about breathing in exercise at the time. A year later, the lecture was published, where he noted: 'the healthy pulmonary system may become a limiting factor to oxygen transport and utilization . . . exercise training elicits functional and structural changes to those organ systems involved in oxygen transport, but the respiratory system remains largely unchanged with training and in turn becomes a weak link'.[8]

I like the sound of Professor Dempsey. You can imagine him in 1985 in the lecture hall, raising some eyebrows and ruffling some feathers among the exercise scientists and physiologists. A touch of Dr Paul Bach-y-Rita and Carlo Rovelli combined, seeking the truth but having to swim upstream to find it. Dempsey's call to arms was for more data, less assumptions, and we seem to be finally starting to make some progress 40 years on. A 2022 review paper suggests that there appears to be a significant shift in the capacity of the respiratory system above 80–85% of VO_2 max.[9] Things naturally go downhill over that intensity if we rely on the auto setting and if we've not trained, as Professor Dempsey described them, our weak links.

When you challenge the way people think about something there is often a lot of push back. No doubt in 1985 Dempsey had his critics, and

I've experienced it first-hand in the elite sporting world. But just like the brain can change and adapt, so can the respiratory system. It can be controlled and therefore changed and trained. It will adapt like any system in the human body to the stresses and challenges we place upon it. It's 40 years since Dempsey challenged the world of science, nearly my entire lifetime. Good news is we're starting to see the light.

Researchers are doing a U-turn on the importance of breathing during exercise, rather than assuming breathing automatically becomes perfectly optimised to meet the demands of our exercise without any training requirement or conscious control from us as runners. The 2022 review agreed with Professor Dempsey noting, 'accumulating evidence strongly suggests that the respiratory system is "underbuilt" for the demands of intense exercise. At exercise around or above 80–85% VO_2 max.'[10]

Going from 'overbuilt' to realising 'underbuilt' is a significant turnaround. Why did we get it so wrong? Why did we make so many assumptions about the complexity of the respiratory system? Something that made a lot of sense to me but was an assumption I had wrong came from an interview with world-renowned running coach Shane Benzie, author of *The Lost Art of Running*, who explained to me, 'We've been given a romantic view of hunter-gathers, that we just run for hours and hours and that we are born and evolved to be able to do that. But it's just not true. The reality is that during a hunt we'd have probably covered about half a marathon and had taken something like eight hours. Hunter-gathers were essentially very good walkers and would run at around a four-hour marathon pace, but weren't running endlessly from dawn till dark.' This challenged what I'd been led to believe, but it made a lot of sense. We aren't adapted to be able to run at higher intensities for hours on end – hence the 80–85% of VO_2 max limit for what the respiratory system seems able to cope with.

At this point, it is probably helpful to know what 80–85% of VO_2 max feels like. For me, as an example from my VO_2 max testing, it is the top end of zone 3 and into zone 4, the threshold where lactate starts to accumulate in the blood as you're moving away from aerobic energy production (zones 2 and 3) into more predominately anaerobic energy production (zones 4 and 5), as the body can't supply oxygen to the working muscles fast enough at that intensity. At this point my heart rate is between 162bpm and 167bpm and I'm running around 14km/hr with 1% gradient, just over 4min/km pace (about 20min for 5km). It's a decent pace for me – close to my 5km PB pace. I'm working hard at that point.

So, it makes sense that if we can find the weak links that limit our breathing, we can look to train them and cope better with demands above 80% of VO_2 max. What are those potential weak links? The previously mentioned study from 2022 cited three mechanisms that limited respiratory performance: 'exercise-induced arterial oxyhaemoglobin desaturation, excessive ventilatory muscle work, and intrathoracic pressure effects on cardiac output'.[11] My rational brain makes sense of that study by asking these logical questions: *can we influence those three mechanisms? Would how we fill our lungs affect the intrathoracic pressure? Could we train the strength of our breathing muscles and the efficiency of how we ventilate?*

These are some big questions. Breathing is less likely to directly influence the oxygen saturation levels of the haemoglobin in our blood, but I have seen in my own testing and research that muscle oxygenation (the relationship between oxygen delivery and consumption at the muscle) with runners can be affected by their breathing. However, the way we ventilate – and the strength of those breathing muscles – is surely something we can train and change.

We've already seen the evidence that elite runners ventilate more efficiently, yet when we feel out of breath, we wish we could get more air in, rather than think about the way we get the air in. Remember Kipchoge coming towards the finish line to break two hours for a marathon, for example. Was he panting and out of breath? No, he was cruising and looking totally in control, relaxed and like he was barely breathing at all.

He's breathing smarter, more efficiently, so he never actually gets out of breath. It's not that he's able to necessarily breathe more and harder than us. A natural assumption is 'more is better' and the commonly used VO_2 max metric plays into this thinking. VO_2 max is the maximum amount of oxygen your body can use during intense exercise in one minute, relative to your bodyweight. It's a metric based on how much you can use rather than how efficiently you use it.

Now don't get me wrong, as exercise intensity increases, the amount of air you need to ventilate increases, but how you get it in may be of more importance than we thought. For example, say I go and have my VO_2 max tested and I hit 50ml/min/kg at a running speed of 18km/hr. I go away and practise breathing techniques that I hope will improve my breathing efficiency and thereby improve my VO_2 max. I come back and retest my VO_2 max, using my practised breathing techniques during the test, but my VO_2 max comes out lower, at say 47ml/kg/min, but the pace I hit my VO_2 max is still 18km/hr. I'm running at the same pace, but my VO_2 max is lower, so we'd say that the breathing techniques didn't help. But let's think about this differently. My VO_2 max is 3ml/kg/min lower, which seems initially a negative, but wait, I'm still running at 18km/hr, the same pace as the original test. So, in fact I'm running at the same pace, but my body is not using or needing as much oxygen. I might be breathing something like 10–15L/min of air less. I was hoping to improve the efficiency of how I was breathing and in this theoretical scenario, that's actually what's happened. Running at the same pace, but breathing less air and needing less oxygen – isn't that the definition of running and breathing more efficiently?

Interestingly, there is an efficiency ratio that can be calculated from the data collected during a VO_2 max test, called 'ventilatory efficiency', yet the majority of researchers don't use or report it because we assume that breathing doesn't affect it. It's the ratio of the total volume of air you are breathing divided by the volume of oxygen your body uses. It's something Professor George Dallam has been researching at Colorado University, which we'll dive deeper into in chapters 4 and 5. For now, I'm simply highlighting that the total amount of oxygen we can use (VO_2 max) might not be as important as how efficiently oxygen is being used.

Remember David Rudisha breaking the 800m world record and taking gold at the London 2012 Olympics with his mouth closed? He was using his nose rather than his mouth predominately. Fair play to Rudisha – he has a decent airway. But nasal breathing will still have restricted the airflow and total ventilation compared with having his mouth wide open. It would make sense he was breathing less air, potentially a slightly lower VO_2 max with his chosen way of breathing. You get gold medals for crossing the line first, not for having the highest VO_2 max. If the guy that came second said, *Yeah, Rudisha might have won the race but I can get more air in through my mouth than he can through his nose*, no one would care! A higher VO_2 max may help you achieve your goal, but it's not the goal in itself. Don't neglect the efficiency of how you're breathing and using oxygen because you're blinkered by focusing purely on how much you can get in or use. Both the amount of oxygen you can use (VO_2 max) and the efficiency of your breathing are important in equal measure.

Efficiency and energy cost

A concept that totally blew my mind related to the efficiency of breathing is that breathing itself has an energy cost. Akin to the chicken and egg conundrum! Your body breathes in order to bring oxygen into the lungs, but in order to breathe, your breathing muscles require oxygen to contract! Professor Dallam explains: 'Oxygen consumption from your breathing muscles can be 15% during running' and if over-breathing, as high as 30%.[12] If I'm more efficient at breathing, I can essentially do it less. If I can do it less, then I spend less energy on it and it uses up less oxygen, which instead can go to the working muscles.

As far back as the 1970s, we've valued the importance of running economy over VO_2 max.[13] Researchers such as David Costill observed elite runners with a similar VO_2 max. He determined that the athlete whose output and performance was best was the athlete who was most economical and used less oxygen at a given running speed, rather than the athlete who used the most oxygen.[14] A 2000 study found that athletes with better running economy outperformed those with a higher VO_2 max.[15] Now, it's important to point out here that running economy isn't specifically about breathing, far from it, it's more about the biomechanics of running and being more efficient in that regard. But it highlights a key point. Using less oxygen at a given pace is a sign of being efficient. We need to be careful in our interpretation of VO_2 max data. Using less oxygen from being more efficient with your running economy is clearly possible – why can't we apply the same principle around being more efficient with how we breathe?

Start breathing like an elite runner

The simplest and most practical thing you can start doing immediately to benefit from more efficient breathing is exactly what I did after just a few weeks of practice for my parkrun 5km PB. Breathing at a slightly slower rate but trying to increase the size and depth of my inhales. Trying to breathe more efficiently, like an elite runner, isn't about trying to ventilate more – it's about doing it smarter.

I couldn't believe the effect of something as simple as breathing slightly slower and slightly deeper than my normal auto. I joined the sub-20-minutes parkrun club. I'd been knocking on the door for over a year, but it was always shut.

> **TRY THIS**
>
> On your next run, follow these steps:
>
> - Simply start by being aware of what your auto breathing feels like when running at a comfortable pace.
> - Become aware of the speed of your breathing and the size and depth of each breath.
> - Keep the pace of your running comfortable as you relax your breathing rate. Rather than specifically trying to slow your breathing down, start by allowing yourself and your breathing to relax.
> - As you relax your chest and abdomen, notice that your breathing slows down naturally. You don't need to breathe as fast as you think you need to, and being relaxed helps this.
> - Finally, as your breathing naturally slows while you relax, try to engage in a deeper and slightly bigger breath as you inhale.
> - Once you become comfortable and relax into this calmer, controlled breathing cycle, you can gradually start to increase your running pace. Try to increase the depth and size of breath rather than just breathing faster to meet the demands of a faster running pace. That's more efficient and what the elite runners do.
>
>

- Relative to what feels normal on auto, you should feel like you're breathing a little slower yet a little bigger and deeper.

I can't promise it will knock a minute off your 5km time straight away, but it's the start of your transformation.

Most runners have got it wrong

Remember I said when crossing the finish line for my parkrun PB I didn't feel like I'd pushed myself, so I didn't think I'd run a good time. Why? Because I wasn't out of breath and that's what I associated (wrongly) with running fast and giving it my best. Why didn't I feel as out of breath? My breathing rate was lower, my breathing was better regulated, and my perceived exertion was lower. Yet I ran a PB!

I was ventilating more like an elite than an amateur, so when I crossed the finish line, like the elites I didn't look or feel particularly out of breath, but I thought that wasn't a good thing. I was more relaxed, more in control and ran faster without realising it. It came as a surprise because I was more relaxed, and I thought I needed to be out of breath to run better or faster. *What an idiot*, I now think! But how many of us have it wrong in our minds what good breathing and running look and feel like?

Ellis Bland, one of the best fell runners in the UK, expressed exactly this to me: most runners have a gross misunderstanding of how to get air in effectively. He went on to explain one of the biggest mistakes he sees runners make: 'If you're gasping for breath, it means you're doing well . . . you shouldn't be gasping for breath, only in a sprint finish or crossing the line.' It's not just me with the misunderstanding of what good breathing is, confusing effort and being out of breath with 'you're doing your best'. Now you might not have an international yoga teacher as your partner like Ellis, but in chapter 8 you'll learn everything you need to know to activate your diaphragm, release its power and ensure you don't make the same mistake.

You can't train breathing without training breathing

Hopefully you're coming round to the idea that just because breathing is automatic, doesn't mean it's optimal. Remember what Professor Dempsey said in 1985: during your training the lung will get left behind as the rest of the system adapts if you aren't specific about training your breathing. Ultimately, you can't train breathing without training breathing.

If we neglect to specifically train our breathing, we leave it to the auto-response, meaning we're more likely to develop compensatory patterns – that's not smarter breathing. Your breathing doesn't necessarily want to change or get better. It wants to maintain homeostasis. Looking at breathing through the lens of a strength and conditioning coach rationalises the fact that your body will adapt to the challenges we place upon it. But that's as long as the challenges are progressive in nature and we allow time for recovery. If you choose to alter your breathing in the right way for certain training sessions for specific outcomes, then we see the body adapt; breathing can and will improve if we train it – just like any other system in the body. But first you have to change your mindset and believe that if you can change it, you can train it and if we can train it, we can make it better.

I said at the start of this chapter we'd unpick some of the assumptions we've made in science about breathing. We've learned that researchers are doing a U-turn and are now recognising the importance of breathing strategies to improve running performance. They've identified that the lungs are, in fact, not built for exercise intensities above 80–85% of VO_2 max, and we've identified that elites cope with higher intensities better than us amateurs, not necessarily by the amount of air they breathe but by how they ventilate it. They do it more efficiently; they regulate their breathing rate with a gradually larger tidal volume and deeper breath. It's more efficient and a calmer breathing rate, allowing them to stay relaxed. In the next chapter we'll look in more detail about why it's more efficient, as well as the other important aspects of breathing that are under our control and therefore trainable, in order to help improve our running.

Key takeaways

- Just because breathing is automatic, doesn't mean it's optimal.
- Breathing can become a weak link if you don't train it specifically.
- We've assumed the lungs are overbuilt but now scientists realise they are underbuilt for intensities greater than 80–85% of VO_2 max.
- Breathing smarter is about doing it more efficiently, rather than just getting more air in. Being able to breathe deeper and increase tidal volume rather than respiratory rate is key to being more efficient.
- More efficient breathing leads to a more controlled, slower breathing rate, which is key to relaxation.

Breath training has opened my eyes to an aspect of performance I thought I understood but had underestimated. It felt like unlocking a new energy reserve. During games, I feel like I can push further through demanding periods. My recovery between sessions and matches has become more efficient, and notably, my sleep quality has improved.

An unexpected benefit was the relief from chronic nasal congestion, making nasal breathing during training and daily life much easier. From my experience, breathwork has significantly enhanced both my athletic performance and overall well-being.

Ollie Thorley, Gloucester and England Rugby

CHAPTER 4

What's the most important thing for runners?

We've learned that elite runners breathe more efficiently than us and now we're going to look at how. We'll uncover what's trainable when it comes to breathing, and we'll use the science underpinning our urge to breathe, so we too can learn and practise to be more relaxed and in control with the power of our breath.

'It will be fast, very fast!'

It's Tuesday evening on 28 May 2024 and rain is hammering down in the Eryri mountains (Snowdonia). It happens to be my 42nd birthday and what better way to celebrate than running up and down a mountain, I thought. I joined around 150 runners who descended on the tiny village of Y Fron. Normally you're more likely to see more sheep hanging around in Y Fron than people. I have no idea what to expect, as the best trail runners in North Wales casually gather for Eryri Harriers Tuesday Evening Series. I've been warned: 'it will be fast, very fast!'

How fast could it be? I thought. We're running up and down Mynydd Mawr, which translates as 'big mountain'. Standing at 673m tall, Mynydd Mawr is no joke, especially as those 673m of elevation happen in less than 1 mile. It's steep. No zigzagging, just up, straight up. *You can't run up all of it, it's too steep*, I thought – another assumption that got me in trouble!

I stood in sidewards rain waiting for 'crazy Mike' to finish the race safety briefing. Once he'd finished laying down the law of the Tuesday night races, suddenly, in a flash, we're off. It was one hell of a pace! As we started the steep climb the pace quite literally took my breath away. I dumped some carbon dioxide, trying to regulate my breathing, and attempted to block out the intense burning sensation screaming from my calves, which had never tried to propel me up a mountain at this type of pace before. Staying relaxed was the last thing on my mind.

Unlike the front runners, I couldn't maintain running the entire way up and had to resort to stints of walking between gingerly jogging. Climbing Mynydd Mawr seemed to go on forever, but the longer it went on, the more I felt like I adjusted to the pace. I kept regulating my breathing with everything I'd been learning. I started to feel gradually better, relative to those around me. As we got closer to the top, you couldn't see much because of the rain, but you knew we were getting close because the front runners were starting to come back down. The first to come down flying past us, barely looking out of breath at all, was a certain Math Roberts.

I decided to count the runners as they came by, 1, 2, 3 . . . soon enough I could see the top. Having been focused on regulating my breathing, I was feeling good, helped by the realisation that the climb would be over in a few minutes, and I started to overtake a few runners on the final part of the climb. It felt good; it felt like the 'breathing secrets' I was implementing were helping. As we turned at the top, I worked out that I was 26th overall, my spirits were high, but I was aware that I'm terrible at the downhills and with this type of rain, I wasn't going to risk anything. I did stack it once in the heather coming down but bounced back up, and five runners flew past me during the one-mile descent. I finished in 31st place in around 45 minutes. Wow, that was around 4.5 miles, with nearly 700m of straight climbing. It blew my mind what the front runners were doing. Had they run the entire way up with no walking at all? They must have done. Math Roberts, the winner, didn't even seem out of breath when he passed us on the way down, finishing in around 30 minutes.

The mountain runners in North Wales (mountain goats, I call them) are made of different stuff, and Math Roberts was a different level. I needed (wanted) to speak to him. We meet in Llanberis to talk running and breathing over coffee. Very quickly the conversation got more exciting, as it turned out that Math, an international runner for Wales, had set all sorts of running records and, most impressively, won everything from a one-mile mountain race to setting ultra-running records. We talked times and numbers. He has run for Wales in the British Fell Running championship and world championships. He has even broken the Paddy Buckley record in 2020 – which covers over 100km, 28,000ft elevation – completing it in an insane 16 hours 37 minutes.

He's run the Ras yr Wyddfa in 1 hour 13 minutes – putting it into perspective, the fastest I've ever got to the top of Yr Wyddfa (Snowdon) is one hour three minutes, so Math and the elite runners would be just cruising in towards the finish having been up and down in the time I can just get to the top! The idea of being fast over one mile but also setting records in ultra-marathons is mind-blowing. Math is a strong runner over any distance: *What was his superpower?* I wondered. *How does he do it?*

Despite his humble nature, Math agrees with me that his ability to win one-mile mountain races as well as set records for ultra-marathons is very unique. My mind flashes back to him running down Mynydd Mawr past me, barely out of breath, and I'm eager to know what his take on breathing is. First, I asked if he ran the entire way up. He sensed my amazement and politely and slightly sheepishly said, 'Yeah it's ok running to the top . . . I think one of the big things is that people don't realise how it's supposed to feel when you're running.'

How does your breathing feel when you are running? How is it meant to feel, are you supposed to feel out of breath? You're supposed to feel out of breath if you've worked really hard, if you're pushing your limits and trying to get better, right? How come that's what makes logical sense and we've all experienced that feeling, yet when someone like Math is running up a mountain he's not out of breath? Or the example of Eliud Kipchoge when he broke the two-hour marathon – he looked at ease coming into the finish line, rather than out of breath. Kipchoge is known for his calm and rhythmic breathing style during races to manage energy, which is more efficient and helps maintain a relaxed state. When you are out of breath, though, you can't relax, but elite runners seem to use their breathing to stay relaxed. There is a relationship with breathing and relaxation that they seem to have got right, which the rest of us seem to have wrong.

Relaxation is key

We're first going to look at this important relationship between breathing and relaxation. We'll unpick the science behind how breathing more efficiently unlocks relaxation and build upon how the elite manage to do it. Research showed amateur runners' tidal volume gets limited much earlier than an elite runner. Why is that important? When the size of your breath is limited, you have to breathe faster, and breathing faster is not relaxing, it's not efficient, so you end up in a vicious downward spiral towards fatigue.

A running coach might have said to you, *breathing should be relaxed and rhythmical.* Yet every time you go out to run you feel out of breath as soon as you start or try to push your pace. Dr Martin Yelling explained that for most runners, one of the biggest barriers to relaxing is daily stress. Your mental state is affected by your breathing because your breathing is interwoven within your ANS, and the speed of your breathing is a key link.

Breathing rate and sympathetic activity (that's the fight or flight response) have a feedback loop; they feed each other. Performance physiotherapist Nigel Beach points out our natural response to running is a stress response, which is faster breathing, feeding more sympathetic activation. Physiologically, higher sympathetic activity is linked to increased muscle tone, especially what's known as flexion tone. Dr Cobb from Z Health Performance, an expert in neurology-based training, explains when you are in fight or flight and the sympathetic nervous system is activated, flexion tone increases to protect the vital organs. A global increase in flexion tone not only stiffens your muscles and makes you feel tense, but it also negatively impacts running posture – you effectively shrink when you tense up, rather than being long, tall and relaxed.

Another key relationship between breathing and your ANS indicates why you're fighting a losing battle when you are breathing fast and feeling out of breath. Your brain has receptors that, when the feeling of being out of breath is strong enough, elicit a primal fear response. The amygdala, a key region of the brain involved in processing fear, is linked with the brain's respiratory centres. When carbon dioxide is increased (like during exercise), if we are particularly sensitive to it, the amygdala activity triggers fear, activating our stress response (sympathetic nervous system), which triggers faster breathing. This has been highlighted in studies where people inhale high enough concentrations of carbon dioxide to trigger panic attacks.[1]

Research suggests that when we are more sensitive to carbon dioxide, we are more prone to fear and anxiety due to the close relationship between the brain's respiratory centres and the amygdala. The faster we run, the more carbon dioxide is produced through cellular respiration. If we are more sensitive to it, we're triggered to breathe faster, making it harder to find that sense of relaxation when running.

During the assessments in chapter 7 you'll learn how to check your own sensitivity to carbon dioxide. And in chapter 10, you'll learn ways to dramatically increase your tolerance of it to help improve your ability to control your breathing rate and stay relaxed.

Finally, being able to control your breathing rate is not only key to staying relaxed and delivering oxygen more efficiently; it also has important implications for your physiology and psychology that will transform your running experience. Cognitive functions that affect focus and your ability to get into a flow state are influenced by the speed of your breathing. Research has shown that slower breathing rates can help reduce sympathetic activity and enhance theta and alpha brainwaves, which promote relaxation and focus – as opposed to faster breathing, which increases beta and gamma brainwaves linked to anxiety.[2] It's physiologically difficult to have a calm, relaxed mind when your sympathetic nervous system is in overdrive and you're breathing fast.

The best athletes in the world who are the masters of controlling their nervous system with their breathing are freedivers. I spoke to world champion freediver Davide Carrera to see what we can learn from them. He said you need to be 'in the present moment, a deep state of meditation'. He explained that if the mind is racing, it's very hard to stay relaxed, as the brain uses up more oxygen. Interestingly the brain is only around 2% of our bodyweight, yet it can use over 20% of our oxygen, vital oxygen that freedivers like Davide want to preserve as they dive down over 100m deep on a single breath, and vital oxygen we, as runners, want to go to our legs.[3] He uses slow breathing to calm the mind and get into a relaxed meditative state before diving. The same principle of the simple, slow, calm breathing that Dr Martin Yelling prescribes the runners he coaches to help them de-stress from daily life before starting their run.

Using breathing to help de-stress from life or calm nerves before a race works because it helps us stay mentally present while lowering the heart rate. You'll learn in chapter 12 how your breathing can be used to help lower the heart rate, improve recovery and reduce fatigue. Even while running, the way we breathe affects the heart, and not just how fast it beats but also the amount of blood the heart can pump per minute, known as your cardiac output. As the heart is situated between the lungs, the pressure changes in the lungs through our breathing have a direct effect on the heart. When we are mechanically breathing optimally (which you'll learn more about chapter 8), it helps increase the ability of the heart to pump more blood per heartbeat (stroke volume), as breathing acts as what's described as a 'respiratory pump', improving venous return to the heart.[4] Cardiac output is a multiple of heart rate and stroke volume. In order to send more blood to working muscles during exercise to deliver vital oxygen, we need to breathe in a way that optimises cardiac output.

We're building up a picture that shows so many of these components to performance are linked and breathing is at the centre.

Finding efficiency

The efficiency of our breathing is a bit of a kingpin in our story because it has a cascade of positive effects on almost everything else when we get it right. An article in 2022 concluded that breathing efficiency is a key player for improving running performance. The researchers stated, 'breathing strategies have the potential to significantly improve ventilatory efficiency and exercise performance'.[5] When you are ventilating more efficiently, you extract more oxygen from each breath, meaning you can do less of it and save energy from the act of breathing itself. This is energy that can go to your legs rather than blood being stolen from your legs when your diaphragm fatigues due to inefficient breathing; this is known as the metaboreflex.

If you're doing your homework, you'll have already made a start on your breathing efficiency by breathing slightly slower with relatively larger and deeper breaths, depending on how fast you are running. To maximise your improvements, we need to understand what's driving our breathing in the first place.

The mechanisms that control our breathing are extremely complex in comparison with how easily breathing automatically happens. If we don't understand what causes us to feel out of breath, it is logical that we are ill-equipped to influence, change or alter it. To understand the mechanisms, we need to dive into some respiratory physiology. Not to blind us with science, but to use science in helping us breathe smarter and become stronger runners.

Basic respiratory physiology

The act of breathing – ventilation – is the movement of air into and out of your lungs. As we inhale, air flows into the lungs via the airway through progressively smaller branches to the tiny air sacs called alveoli. How we fill these little air sacs is essential to breathing efficiently, which we'll learn by the end of the chapter. The alveoli are very important, as the exchange of oxygen and carbon dioxide takes place here through the membrane wall, which is just one cell thick to allow for easy diffusion. When blood arrives at the lungs, it is lower in oxygen, as our tissues have used it, and higher in carbon dioxide, as our tissues have created it. At the lungs, oxygen diffuses from the alveoli into the blood, and carbon dioxide diffuses in the other direction. The surface area of the lungs is huge, due to the number of alveoli. If you stretched them out flat, the total surface area of your lungs would be about half a tennis court (please don't do that though, or you'll be dead!). The surface area is huge, the membrane wall is just one cell thick, so it's perfectly designed for diffusion to happen easily.[6]

At school we typically get taught a drastically overly simplified exchange of oxygen in and carbon dioxide out. It leads to misconceptions about what is good and what is bad; typically we see oxygen as good and carbon dioxide as the bad guy. We also fall into a trap that simply more is better when it comes to breathing. In fairness, it's logical to think that if you breathe more air in, you'll get more oxygen in and have more energy. Rather than only thinking 'how much', we need to also think about how efficiently we're able to do it, including both how the oxygen is coming in and how well our body manages carbon dioxide.

The air we breathe in the atmosphere has been stable for around 550 million years.[7] That's a long time and we're pretty used to it by now. It's only around 20.9% oxygen and around 0.04% carbon dioxide. The majority is nitrogen, which is around 78%. However, the air we breathe out is around 16% oxygen and 4–5% carbon dioxide.[8] Your body uses around 25% of the oxygen you inhale, meaning it breathes out around 75% of oxygen you just inhaled, and creates around 100 times more carbon dioxide than it inhales. Hold on, 75% of the oxygen you breathe in, you breathe out – *what do you mean?* Your body only uptakes about 25% of the oxygen in each breath. That's at rest. *I bet when you're exercising, your body uses all that oxygen?* Nope. Depending on how efficiently you breathe, you will extract more or less oxygen from each breath. Newsflash: if you breathe really inefficiently, you might get more air in your lungs, but you extract less oxygen as a percentage from each breath and therefore have to keep breathing more.

To understand how to be more efficient with our breathing, we need to understand a few more basics about breathing mechanics, the lungs and what's controlling our breathing.

The mechanical aspect of breathing is simply about increasing the size or volume in the thorax (chest cavity), which decreases your internal pressure. As air, like any gas, moves from pressures of high to low. When you increase the internal volume (by expanding the thorax), you decrease the pressure relative to the air pressure outside, and air is drawn in. That's breathing, in a nutshell. Now, like any movement pattern it can be performed more or less efficiently – through optimal movement patterns, with good ribcage positioning and diaphragm function (you'll learn how to optimise in chapters 8 and 9), or through compensatory movement patterns involving more of your accessory breathing muscles. It can take more or less energy to perform, depending on how you do it. If you do it efficiently, you don't have to do it as much.

Just as we don't use all of the oxygen in each breath, we don't use all of our lungs. The faster you are triggered to breathe, the harder it is to fill the lungs efficiently, as well as the amount you can get in. Your total lung capacity is the maximum amount of air in the lungs after a full inhalation at rest. But you can't use all of this because there is always a certain amount of air left in the lungs at rest, called functional residual capacity, because if the lungs fully emptied, they'd collapse in on themselves. At the end of a maximal exhale, this remaining amount of air is the residual capacity, which is typically around one litre. Just because you might have a total lung capacity of six litres, it doesn't mean you can use all six litres. The amount you can potentially use would be six litres (total lung capacity) minus what's left in the lungs (residual capacity), which is about one litre. This means you have a maximum of five litres to play with, known as forced vital capacity.[9] During exercise it drops further, as you don't have all the time in the world to take the biggest forced breath you possibly can. As we've alluded to, the faster you breathe, the more you restrict the lungs because you just don't have the time to fill them up efficiently.

Your speed of breathing and how much air you get into your lungs dictates the total volume of air you're breathing, known as minute ventilation (V_E). If your tidal volume (V_T) is restricted, then you have to breathe faster (respiratory rate, RR) in order to breathe more air during exercise.

$$V_E = RR \times V_T$$

At rest, an average male exchanges approximately 0.5 litres (400ml for females) of air per breath (tidal volume), 12 times/minute, providing a minute ventilation rate of around six litres of air/minute.[10] As we start exercising, ventilation increases to match the required oxygen uptake needed to oxygenate our muscles adequately and remove carbon dioxide. At lower levels of exercise intensity, we typically see both RR and

V_T increase. But as we learned in the last chapter, elite athletes don't necessarily ventilate more air as they get challenged by exercise; it's the *way* they ventilate and their ability to increase their tidal volume – even all the way to exhaustion. On the other hand, amateur runners are often restricted by their ability to increase the size of their breath. This means they only have the option to increase the speed of breathing, leading to shallow upper chest-dominant breathing – reported to have negative effects on performance, such as 'increased flow limitation, workload of breathing, hyperventilation, and postural instability'.[11]

What's controlling our breathing?

How do we get better control of breathing rate? We need to look now at what's actually stimulating us to breathe, to learn how to control it better. It's not as simple as you might think; it's certainly not just about oxygen. Carbon dioxide, how your lungs and diaphragm stretch, and our perception of breathing and effort during exercise are all key players too.

The respiratory centres in your brain stem don't just track oxygen levels to control ventilation. They get feedback from several different sources at the lungs, in the blood and even your mind, relating to how you think you're supposed to breathe. As oxygen is so important and vital to life, there are receptors in the body that detect when levels are low in the transporting blood and muscle cells. There are things in our muscles that detect hypoxia (low oxygen) when exercising, but these are not chemoreceptors as in the blood and brain stem. Hypoxia-inducible-factor-1α (HIF-1α) is an intracellular oxygen sensor helping to regulate oxygen in the muscle along with help from myoglobin, an intracellular oxygen reservoir. Muscle afferent nerves (group III & IV), send feedback to the brain by indirectly detecting low oxygen through metabolic waste products, such as lactate and hydrogen ion accumulation.

However, because there is the time gap between breathing and oxygen reaching the blood from the lungs, circulating the whole body and reaching the tissues takes around 16 seconds. That delay would result in fluctuations of oxygen levels that would be dangerous, as oxygen is so important to every cell in our body. Therefore, other inputs play vital roles in driving our breathing to ensure that we have oxygen in abundance within our blood and supplied to our muscles.

Carbon dioxide travels in the opposite direction to oxygen. It's made in the cells, transported in the blood to the lungs, diffused through the alveoli and exhaled. Part of the transportation of carbon dioxide in the blood creates a pH change, as 65% is converted to carbonic acid (which separates into bicarbonate and hydrogen ion), increasing acidity, which is known as respiratory acidosis. This is important because the blood levels of carbon dioxide affects respiratory acidosis (increase in hydrogen ions) – a key component of fatigue as Dr Anna Robins, who conducted my VO_2 max testing as part of my research at Salford University, explained: 'the accumulation of hydrogen ions is one of the things that interferes with muscle contractile elements and leads to muscle fatigue'.

During higher-intensity exercise, as well as from respiratory acidosis, with the production of lactate as a result of anaerobic energy production (without oxygen), we also see an increase in acidity (hydrogen ions) from what's known as metabolic acidosis. In his book *Hypoventilation Training*, French researcher Xavier Woorons explains how carbon dioxide can also limit the release of lactate from the muscle cells to the blood.[12] So not only do increased carbon dioxide and lactate both increase acidosis and contribute to fatigue, they are also related. How our muscles and blood deal with and buffer the acidity created from both carbon dioxide and lactate production is something that Xavier Woorons has shown we can train and improve. He uses a unique breath-holding technique, which you'll learn about in chapter 10, potentially increasing your body's ability to tolerate lactate and its ability to remove it.

The way your body clears carbon dioxide is through your exhalation. How well you can tolerate levels of carbon dioxide in your lungs and blood, therefore, has a significant impact on your ability to control your breathing. At first impression, it seems like our science teacher at school was right: carbon dioxide makes our blood more acidic and we need to breathe it out – it's a waste gas. But it's not as simple as that, and we need to start making friends with carbon dioxide. It's a powerful gas that needs to be regulated and kept in balance.

Carbon dioxide plays vital roles within the bloodstream as it's transported from the tissues to the lungs. It helps with circulation as a vasodilator (so blood vessels open up), manages blood pressure regulation (through baroreceptors) and it even plays a key role in the release of oxygen from the blood, known as the Bohr effect. It's not a new concept: in 1904 Christian Bohr identified the role carbon dioxide has on the pH of the blood and the resulting impact on oxygen delivery from the blood to the tissues. Essentially, it helps us transport oxygen in the blood and release it from the red blood cells.

It fascinates me that the thing the body creates more of during exercise (carbon dioxide) is what helps to improve the things we need to happen when we exercise. We need more blood circulation, more oxygen delivery and we need to breathe a larger volume of air (in proportion with our metabolic demands, remember). Guess what, increasing carbon dioxide levels helps with all of that. It's like the body knows what it needs, and it uses what it creates to give it what it needs. It dramatically changes the narrative around carbon dioxide. It stops it being labelled as a waste gas we need to get rid of as we start to understand that we need to recalibrate our relationship with it.

It's also one of the components that plays a role in what's driving our urge to breathe and our sensation of feeling out of breath. It's complex to understand all the mechanisms that are driving it, but carbon dioxide is part of the puzzle. We'll look now at how it affects our urge to breathe, what other mechanisms are responsible for feeling out of breath and how they are processed in the brain.

The brain stem is made up of three parts: mid-brain, pons and medulla. The respiratory centres are located in the pons and medulla. Interestingly, the two components that control our ventilation – respiratory rate and tidal volume – are controlled by these two different parts of the brain stem – the medulla and pons, respectively.

We have many different types of receptors. The two most important for runners are chemoreceptors and mechanoreceptors. They all feed into the respiratory centres in the brain stem, known as central chemoreceptors. Within the medulla we also have the pre-Bötzinger complex, which is responsible for the rhythm of our breathing. Other receptors outside the brain include peripheral chemoreceptors at the neck and heart and mechanoreceptors located in the lungs, which all provide vital feedback via cranial nerves to the respiratory centre in the brain to help it modulate our breathing, rate, depth and rhythm.[13]

The central chemoreceptors primarily sense pH changes caused by changes in blood carbon dioxide levels. As carbon dioxide diffuses across the blood–brain barrier, the chemoreceptors sense the change in pH (increased acidity) and send sensory input to the brain to stimulate an increase in ventilation. This helps exhale more carbon dioxide in order to regulate blood pH, which needs to remain between 7.35 and 7.45. Your inhale dictates your exhale, so if you are stimulated to inhale more air, you will also exhale more air and, in doing so, will lower carbon dioxide levels in the lungs and blood and restore pH levels.[14]

The peripheral chemoreceptors include the carotid and aortic bodies, located in the neck and near the heart, respectively. They send information to the respiratory centres in the brain via nerves. However, they have less of an influence on our urge to breathe, comprising around 15% of the stimuli for respiration. 'In healthy individuals, the respiratory centre is more sensitive to rising carbon dioxide sensed by central chemoreceptors than decreasing oxygen levels. Oxygen runs the respiratory centre only when there is severe hypoxemia.'[15]

Finally, we have stretch and pressure receptors called mechanoreceptors, found in the smooth muscle of the walls in the airways, trachea, lungs and pulmonary vessels. They send sensory feedback to the respiratory centres about lung volume, airway stretch and vascular congestion via the vagus nerve. These receptors help sense stretch in the lungs to prevent overinflation to protect them, known as the Hering-Breuer inflation reflex. They also provide information about the size of inhalation stretch.[16] Mechanoreceptors are also found in the diaphragm and chest wall, which provide information to the respiratory centres in the brain about the movement of the diaphragm and the expansion of the ribcage, and are believed to be responsible for the sensation of fullness at the top of a breath.

Integration of receptor input

All of these different sensory receptors provide valuable feedback to the brain, which then modulates how much air we breathe in any given moment by controlling the speed (respiratory rate), rhythm, size and depth (tidal volume) of our breathing.

There has been some interesting research to try and decipher if any one variable is more important. For example, you'd think that if you paralysed the breathing muscles and increased carbon dioxide by holding the breath, they'd still feel the urge to breathe based on high levels of carbon dioxide. However, a study titled 'The Effect of Muscular Paralysis Induced by Curarization on Breath Holding in Normal Subjects' demonstrated this wasn't the case. It found that 'the distressing sensation normally experienced during breath-holding was absent' and there was no uncomfortable out-of-breath sensation felt in the chest.[17] We'd expect the urge to breathe to still be present regardless of the temporary paralysis of the breathing muscles, but this wasn't the case. This suggests that the breathing muscles and perhaps the lungs themselves are what causes the majority of the uncomfortable sensation when we feel out of breath.

A further study explored differences in pressure changes in the lungs during both inhalation and exhalation, finding only a minor contribution from chemoreceptors in the detection of abnormal blood levels of carbon dioxide, compared with a more significant effect from pressure changes. They observed that the discomfort in breathing was limiting exercise performance and the pressure changes in the lungs affected those sensations more than changes in carbon dioxide, highlighting the importance of the mechanoreceptors in the lungs. They also noted that the exhale was also very important in the 'overall perception of difficulty in breathing in healthy subjects during exercise'.[18]

We'll learn in chapters 9 and 11 how we can use exhalations to our advantage with a little secret breathing hack based on this principle to help us feel less out of breath when we are pushing our limits!

The final piece of the puzzle that drives our urge to breathe is related to the perception of difficulty. It makes me think back to the comment from Math Roberts about runners not knowing how breathing is meant to feel. If we don't know what it's supposed to feel like, our perception of those sensations may well affect our emotional state and psychology.

Martin McPhilimey is a respiratory and sleep clinical scientist who places great emphasis on emotions and breathing. He explained in our interview, 'breathing itself is informed by prior beliefs... the brain models certain breathing behaviours and is good at predicting the right way to breathe in a given situation'. He believes that breathing is a 'behaviour, a conditioned response in how we feel in our emotional state'. A 2009 study states that the 'respiratory sensation is generated by corollary discharges of the central motor commands to the respiratory muscles', which is separate to any feedback from the lungs, muscle or heart.[19] As Martin McPhilimey suggests, our emotional state creates a response in our breathing that is not linked to chemoreceptors or mechanoreceptors. Our perception of how out of breath we feel when we're running can signal to our respiratory muscles to breathe faster. Perceived exertion is also affected by how the diaphragm contracts and fatigues. Another study noted that perceived effort increases 'at a faster rate with the high pressure-short duty cycle pattern of contraction'. Strong, fast contractions of the diaphragm rather than slower contractions significantly increased effort perception despite muscle fatigue being relatively equal.[20]

A further study highlighted the sensation of feeling out of breath has two distinct sensations: 'effort or work of breathing' and 'air hunger', with the air hunger sensation being described as more discomfort than 'effort'.[21] The study observed that these sensations can occur simultaneously or independently and noted air hunger sensations correlated with carbon dioxide chemosensitivity and effort/work sensation correlated with respiratory muscle and lung mechanoreceptors. Interestingly, they concluded from this that increases in tidal volumes relieve air hunger.

This is absolute gold when you relate it to what elite runners already do. They regulate the speed of their breathing by increasing their tidal volume (which activates the mechanoreceptors), reducing the sensation of air hunger. They feel less out of breath; hence they can relax. The perception of effort and air hunger for an amateur runner will always be higher until we improve our tolerance to carbon dioxide, our breath control and mechanically expand our ribcage to breathe in a more efficient way by increasing tidal volume, rather than simply breathing faster.

Our breathing rate is so critical to our performance and a 'marker of physical effort', that research now acknowledges that our breathing rate is a more reliable marker of RPE (rate of perceived exertion) than other physiological markers usually used, such as heart rate and blood lactate levels.[22]

Our breathing rate and perception of breathing sensations, our psychology, chemosensitivity to carbon dioxide and the mechanoreceptors' feedback to the brain are all potentially linked. The good news is we can train them all to change how we physically and mentally respond to breathing during exercise. That might change both our performance and our perception of effort and fatigue levels.

Breathing more efficiently

Let's conclude this section with how we can actually breathe more efficiently, which means getting a greater proportion of oxygen to your alveoli so more can be extracted per breath. The efficiency of your breathing, ventilatory efficiency, is calculated as the ratio of the volume of oxygen your body extracted (VO_2) divided by total ventilation (V_E).

$$\text{Ventilatory Efficiency} = VO_2 / V_E$$

Essentially, if you are more efficient at breathing, you have less oxygen in your exhalation because your body has been able to extract and use more from each breath. Unfortunately, as part of the overlooked nature of breathing, many scientists I've spoken to are dismissive of the idea that the ventilatory efficiency is something that breathing could alter, as it's deemed to be an autonomic function outside of our control.

One study suggested that ventilatory efficiency may be an inherent characteristic, independent of 'fitness level, anthropometric profile, age or the ergometer used for testing'.[23] However, the study didn't actually assess whether breathing differently could alter ventilatory efficiency. They tested subjects doing different types of exercises and, of course, each subject just breathed how they would normally breathe. It didn't really prove anything other than people have a 'normal' way of breathing which they take with them into all types of exercise.

Not all researchers are built the same. Every now and again, someone breaks the rules and we change the way we see things. In 2018 the first study was published demonstrating how our ventilation during exercise affects oxygen efficiency. When I found out one of the researchers from that study was not just a professor but also a triathlete, I thought we'd hit the jackpot. Not just someone with theories in a lab, but someone who had a lived experience of it. Not only was he a professor at Colorado State University and a competitive triathlete himself, he's also worked as a coach for the US Olympic triathlon team. This is a researcher who doesn't just know the science of it – he's lived and breathed it. Meet Professor George Dallam.

Professor Dallam is an advocate of nasal breathing, but don't get too hung up on that now, as we cover the nose v mouth debate in the next chapter. In his 2018 study they took five males and five females who'd practised nasal breathing during running for at least six months and performed VO_2 max tests comparing mouth breathing and nasal-only breathing. Their nasal breathing was indeed more efficient than their mouth breathing 'with superior physiological economy and ventilatory efficiency'. They breathed over 20% slower and needed 22% less air to produce the same output with no loss in VO_2 max.[24]

Astonishing! That makes you ask a few questions, right? Me too, and I did – I jumped on a call with Professor Dallam as soon as I could. He explained that with nasal breathing, there is more time for oxygen diffusion at the lungs due to the slower breathing rate, meaning that more oxygen can be absorbed with each breath. Again, this highlights the importance of regulating speed of breathing for runners. Controlling the speed of breathing and the size or depth of each breath can also improve alveolar ventilation.

Alveolar ventilation refers to the amount of air actually reaching the tiny air sacs called alveoli, rather than the total amount of air you breathe.

That's because around 150ml of air is in your trachea and branching airways, where the exchange of oxygen and carbon dioxide can't happen.[25] For every breath, when running and breathing with a tidal volume of say two litres, only around 1.85 litres (2L - 150ml) of air gets to the alveoli, where gas exchange takes place. The unused air in the tracheal dead volume or pulmonary dead space means that the faster you breathe, potentially the more air you 'waste' in this dead space.[26] A 2022 study suggested this as a variable that could modify ventilatory efficiency.[27] Essentially, if you are able to maintain control of a better breathing rate, and proportionally increase the tidal volume, just as the elite runners do, you create 'more oxygen-rich breaths' as more air can reach the alveoli with each breath.[28]

Slower breathing also gives us an opportunity to mechanically ventilate more efficiently, too. The shape of the lungs means that towards the bottom we have a greater mass and density of the alveoli. Fast breathing means there isn't time for air to be drawn low into the lungs – it pumps from the upper chest in what we described as shallow breathing. This creates a vicious cycle. As we are breathing less efficiently, we need to do it more, which is harder work for your accessory breathing muscles, and therefore your perception of effort is high and you feel out of breath.

When you are breathing more efficiently, with an increase in tidal volume, you don't have to do it as much. Your perception of effort is lower and, importantly, you can relax into your running. A great example of this was with an amateur runner Des Hughes, who immediately felt the difference of trying to breathe in a more efficient fashion when running, by controlling the speed of breathing with bigger and deeper breaths. His muscle oxygenation when tested was more stable and he told me, 'It felt easier running up hill, it felt a bit different at first but when I relaxed it felt better.'

How you breathe can also protect the lungs

A very important population of runners that nasal breathing can have a massive effect on is those with asthma. Up to 70% of the population can be affected by exercise-induced asthma during sports, and our noses can provide protection.[29] Remember Tess, the highly competitive ultra-marathon runner? In her words her asthma was 'pretty bad at the moment', but having done some work on her nasal breathing and breathing mechanics, just a week later I received a text: 'I forgot my asthma inhaler at the race I did on Saturday and managed to not need it through just focusing on breathing better at the start.'

Essentially, the nose helps to protect the airways and the lungs. It marks the start of your immune system, with an important gas produced inside the nose called nitric oxide, which is antiviral, antifungal, anti-everything! The nasal cavity also warms, moistens and humidifies the air, which stops the airway getting dry and irritated and leading to inflammation and narrowing of the airway when cold, unconditioned air hits the back of the throat with mouth breathing. The effect can be quite astonishing, as Tess found out.

> **TRY THIS**
>
> **Feel the effect of carbon dioxide**
> You can put into practice what we've learned quite easily. Try this to feel the immediate effect of combining the build-up of carbon dioxide with stimulation of the stretch receptors in your lungs and diaphragm on your urge to breathe.
>
> Take a normal breath in and out, and then hold your breath and time how long it takes you to feel that first urge to breathe (not your maximum breath-hold time). Then have a short break and compare that to first taking 5–10 big, deep and full inhalations and exhalations to 'blow off' more carbon dioxide than normal and stretch those mechanoreceptors at the top of your inhale.
>
> After your final full exhalation, pause and hold your breath and time how long it takes for you to feel that first urge to breathe. You'll notice that immediately after lowering your carbon dioxide levels by 'blowing it off' and stimulating those mechanoreceptors with larger inhalations, your urge to breathe comes later than just a few moments ago.
>
> Building up our tolerance to carbon dioxide and being able to mechanically expand the ribcage, fill the lungs and engage the diaphragm could surely give us better control of breathing when ventilation demand increases while running.

When and where to practise?

To use what we've learned, we obviously need to practise. You can practise breathing while sat down or lying down, but it might not help your breathing while running. A 2020 study noted that although three weeks of static breathing exercises improved some functions of breathing, it didn't affect running economy and exercise performance.[30]

However, a more recent study in 2023 suggests potential benefits of static breathing exercises on running performance, as it may improve ventilation and respiratory control leading to improved running velocities, at a similar perception of effort.[31] In my experience, though, if you want to improve your breathing during running, you need to work on your breathing when running. A sigh of relief, I'm sure. You might not be interested in long breath-focused meditation sessions – you want to be out pounding the streets or on the trails, which are the best places to practise your breathing.

The remaining chapters in this book detail how to practise specific breathing techniques during running and training to breathe smarter and run stronger. You can start straight away with the most important factor we've highlighted so far: the speed of your breathing affects your efficiency and your relaxation. Simply being aware of your breathing naturally starts to slow it down, and until you are aware of your breathing, you won't be able to do anything about changing it. Your warm-up (if you do one) is a great time to be a bit more aware of your breathing as you aren't fully into your running yet, so you can focus on something else (your breath) without it disrupting your run.

Potential immediate impact on performance

Previous research has highlighted the impact of training breathing mechanics, carbon dioxide tolerance with breath-holds and nasal-only breathing, which may improve overall aerobic output and lower fatigue in longer training sessions.[32] It was also noted that 'increasing tolerance to carbon dioxide and improving breathing mechanics may help reduce anxiety', which is particularly helpful in managing the stress of intense training sessions or performance anxiety around races and running events.

In practice, I've seen these techniques have an immediate impact on performance, for example, Olympic athlete and England Rugby player Alex Matthews. After the initial assessments (*see* chapter 7) we identified areas of her ribcage that were restricting her breathing, we assessed breathing and muscle oxygenation in an incremental exercise test to see how well she was oxygenating her muscles, as well as how efficiently she was ventilating, during the exercise test. After mobilising the ribcage, practising how to mechanically ventilate more efficiently as well as activating the diaphragm, we retested.

Astonishingly, she managed to increase her tidal volume from 2.38 litres to 2.57 litres, an 8% improvement. This led to over 50% improvement in total ventilation per minute and meant she lasted 15% longer in the test. She also hit a higher output (6% increase), with the same heart rate and muscle oxygenation. Smarter breathing improved her performance intensity, output and duration. Not surprisingly, she felt better and noted that it felt easier and she was more in control.

These same performance improvements for your running are waiting for you. Your breathing is the invitation.

In my experience, understanding some respiratory physiology is helpful in learning how and why these different breathing techniques can transform your running. I hope it's been helpful for you too.

We've learned the kingpin is the efficiency of your breathing. We know that the speed of breathing is essential for that, and it provides a cascade of positive effects on your physiology and psychology. We know relaxation is the most important thing in the acute act of running, and how breathing efficiency and rate directly impact it. Later you'll also learn how to equip yourself with breathing techniques to use in training to make long-term adaptations that will ultimately change your auto setting for the better.

Key takeaways

- The speed of our breathing has a cascade of effects not just on our physical performance but also our mental state and psychology, which influences our perception of effort during exercise and ability to relax.
- The brain receives a multitude of inputs from the body creating our urge to breathe: notably, sensitivity to carbon dioxide and mechanoreceptors, which are trainable and allow us to control our breathing more easily and reduce our perception of effort.
- More control over our breathing rate allows for a slower and deeper breath, which is more efficient, as it allows more time for diffusion at the lungs, improving alveolar ventilation.
- Faster breathing rates increase the fight or flight response and flexion tone, stiffening your muscles, restricting your running form and ability to increase tidal volume.

Training with Jacko has been a game changer. His practical, no-nonsense approach made breathwork immediately applicable to my life and training. Jacko doesn't just teach techniques – he constantly challenges you to apply them in real-world scenarios, pushing the boundaries of what you think breathwork can do.

As I train for my first ultra-trail race, his teachings have become essential. Using breath-holds in my warm-ups, while nasal breathing during long runs keeps my effort efficient and sustainable. Post-run down-regulation techniques are key to accelerating my recovery. Despite increasing my weekly mileage, I'm bouncing back quicker than ever.

→

> Jacko's energy, clarity and support have made this journey not only more effective but also more enjoyable. Thank you, Jacko, for your guidance, your friendship, and for helping me breathe better, run stronger, and recover faster.
>
> **Ciaran Avitabile, runner and breathing coach**

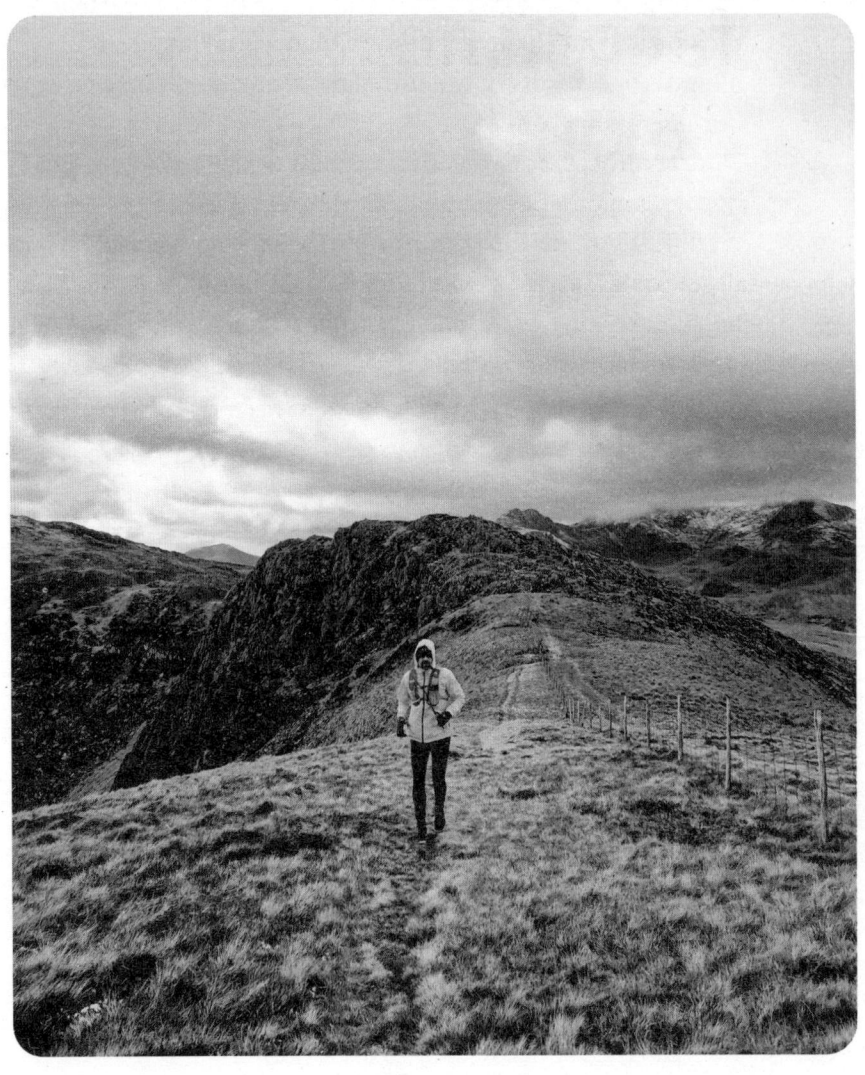

CHAPTER 5

Which hole in your face? The nose v mouth debate

Before we all get our knickers in a twist because we assume nasal breathing while running is ridiculous, if not impossible, let's see what some experts say. Here, we'll look at why the latest research suggests incorporating nasal breathing into some of our training can transform our performance and even protect our heart.

The danger of closing the big hole

The debate of which hole in your face you should be breathing through during running has been a hot topic of discussion. When you first try nasal breathing, you either love it or you hate it. In typical Jacko fashion, when I heard about the potential benefits, I threw myself into it 'whole hog'. Everyone's starting point and initial capacity with their nose is unique to them. My starting point was a few years after recovering from the traumatic brain injury that ended my professional rugby career. I was back to running, the pace was very slow, but I didn't care, I was just happy to be moving again. Despite the slow pace I found nasal breathing very hard initially. It felt uncomfortable, my breathing mechanics were still all upper chest and anytime I ran over 5km, I'd have neck and shoulder pain.

I now realise that was triggered by overworking my accessory breathing muscles, as I was sucking up with my nose, using it like a vacuum cleaner rather than like an actual nose. But I didn't know any better.

Time passed and some important adaptations occurred and nasal breathing started to do wonders for my running. When I got it right, it felt great at a comfortable pace, like I could go forever. I signed up for a three-day ultra, which – assuming nasal breathing would help me run 216km – was a mistake! I tried to keep it nasal on day three, which helped me regulate and seemingly come 'back from the dead'. But I'd reduced the simplicity of breathing to just closing the bigger hole in my face and using the two smaller ones instead. I was ignorant to think that breathing a certain way would make up for the inexperience and lack of conditioning for such a multi-day event.

I'd not done enough homework. On average I'd barely manage 20km a week in my training yet managed to scrape myself to the finish line. Would more training allow for more adaptation? Would increasing my carbon dioxide tolerance, ventilating efficiently with better mechanics help? Or was nasal breathing not all that it's cracked up to be?

Nose v mouth

It's helpful to have a better understanding of the anatomy of the nose, mouth and the airway to help make informed decisions about breathing.

The nose is smack bang in the middle of your face, taking up a huge amount of 'prime real estate' – it makes sense that it must be pretty important. If I think rationally about it, it must do more than just smell, because you can survive many things and challenges in life without being able to smell. Maybe its purpose is something as important as breathing?

Breathing expert Patrick McKeown has now identified 33 different functions of the nose that the mouth doesn't possess. Some of those functions include humidifying, warming, moistening and filtering the air. It has a protective effect on the airway and lungs. It has a different effect on your ANS than mouth breathing, supporting cognitive function through the olfactory nerve. Yet mouth breathing at rest has been linked with dysfunctional breathing patterns, upper respiratory tract infections, rhinitis and asthma. It's now widely accepted that the nose is the 'primary point of entry and exit' of the airway during healthy breathing at rest, but it's less clear what's healthy or optimal during exercise.[1]

I've had the pleasure of learning from and working with Patrick McKeown at the Oxygen Advantage, and I asked him why, if nasal breathing is better than mouth breathing during running, does almost every runner breathe with their mouth open? 'It's very simple. It's easier. The air hunger is less. Essentially you don't feel as "out of breath."' Patrick goes on to explain: 'Poor breathing is inefficient, it's un-economical, you're wasting energy and it can affect your mind. Poor breathing can be overcome by willpower and physical training adaptations but at what cost? However, once adapted to nasal breathing you can breathe more efficiently, so you don't need to breathe as hard for a given intensity.'

The size of the nose is one of three key factors affecting your nasal breathing ability at different running intensities. My mind flashes back to David Rudisha setting that 800m world record with his mouth seemingly closed – could the size of his nose mean it's possible for him but not someone like me?

Everyone's noses are different shapes and sizes. As Patrick points to his nose and nods at me and my small narrow nose, he asks, 'Rudisha would be breathing maybe 150L/min. Could you ventilate that amount of air with your nose?' No chance. In fact, during my VO_2 max testing I managed to achieve 80 litres/minute as a maximum before I had to open my mouth. Patrick makes a clear point: not all noses are made equal. The size and shape of your nose plays a large role in your ability to ventilate the required amount of air with it. And we are stuck with the nose we were born with. Deviated septums and broken noses can also affect how much air you can ventilate nasally. I work with many international rugby players and mixed martial arts (MMA) fighters who regularly have their noses bashed in, and there are still things we do to help them with their nasal breathing despite structural challenges.

The size and shape of your nose and how much air you can ventilate with it surely impacts the intensity or pace of running we can manage nasally, which is something we cover later. First, if nasal breathing is more efficient, why has it been so badly overlooked in the research?

Researchers give us only one option in testing

A number of the experts and researchers I've spoken to have all raised an important point about studying nasal breathing. To measure blood gases and ventilation dynamics in a laboratory setting, we have to wear a mask. A mask that was ultimately designed with the assumption that during exercise the subject would be mouth breathing. The masks used do allow for and capture nasal breathing, but anyone who's worn one in a VO_2 max test, for example, will know what I mean when I say it feels a little restrictive and even claustrophobic on the nose.

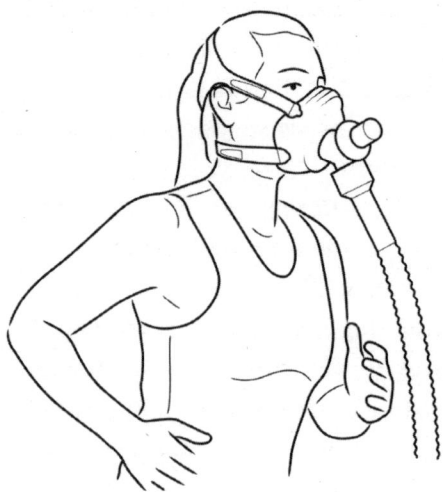

An exercise-test mask can feel claustrophobic on your nose

You're more likely to mouth breathe during exercise with one of those masks on, especially if you aren't aware of the difference between the nose and mouth. Research is now starting to acknowledge this and recommends caution in exercise physiology testing with spiroergometry masks (see above) in view of their detrimental effects on breathing.

Studies recommend that more natural settings are used to investigate nasal breathing with minimally invasive equipment.[2]

It's a challenge, though, as it's currently very difficult to capture and analyse someone's ventilation outside of the laboratory setting in a 'natural' way. We do now have portable devices but having a mask stuck to your face doesn't feel normal when you are running outside. That said, Professor George Dallam has been successful in the laboratory setting, despite those challenges for nasal breathing, to prove it can be better than mouth breathing for running. His 2020 review paper states, 'a significant body of evidence also unanimously illustrates the concept that nasal breathing results in better ventilatory efficiency than oral/oronasal breathing during exercise, which may also result in an improvement in physiological economy.'[3]

At the crux of the benefits of nasal breathing during running seems to be that it's more efficient. I ask Professor Dallam what 'being more efficient' means when it comes to the nose and whether it takes time for the nose to be more efficient with practice. Nasal breathing has greater ventilatory efficiency, right out of the box,' he explains. 'Basically, you'll breathe less to create the same oxygenation when you are breathing nasally regardless of whether you've adapted yet or not, so long as you can ventilate sufficiently for the given exercise intensity.'

In his book *The Nasal Breathing Paradox During Exercise*, Professor Dallam notes that many studies support the benefits of nasal breathing during steady state submaximal exercise (not just his research), as it creates 'a lower respiration rate, lower ventilation, lower ventilatory equivalent for both oxygen and carbon dioxide'. This results in improved ventilatory efficiency, slower breathing and less air ventilated when nasal breathing compared to mouth breathing, but still oxygenating sufficiently.[4]

All of the benefits of efficient breathing appear to happen naturally when you use your nose. In one study, when breathing nasally with the same tidal volume at the same workload, compared with mouth breathing, subjects had less oxygen and more carbon dioxide in their exhalations.[5] This indicates that the body uses more oxygen per breath (when nasal breathing), as there was less oxygen in the exhale, and tolerates higher levels of carbon dioxide, as it can't leave through the nose as fast as it can through the mouth.

What is it about the nose that means more oxygen is extracted per breath, improving ventilatory efficiency? According to Professor Dallam, the resistance your breathing muscles have to overcome when nasal breathing is due to the smaller holes. This means air enters the lungs more forcefully, thereby increasing pressure in the lungs, helping increase the distribution of air within the lungs and the diffusion of oxygen from the lungs into the blood. The increased levels of nitric oxide in the nose as a vasodilator also helps increase pulmonary blood flow.

Increased resistance appears to improve diaphragm recruitment and assists air more forcefully and deeper into the lungs. Lower in the lungs there is a greater density of alveoli and more blood (due to gravity). Breathing slower into those lower regions helps reduce air lost in dead space, optimising alveolar ventilation.

This increased resistance is a double-edged sword, however. As I experienced, it's not all sunshine and rainbows when you shut your mouth and run. Increased resistance is uncomfortable, like you're working harder, and it can feel restrictive. Does the nose limit the amount of air we breathe? Professor Dallam explained that although we ventilate less with nasal breathing (~20%), oxygenation is still as good. The blood and muscles still receive similar oxygen levels because oxygen extraction at the lungs is more efficient, so you don't need as much air when you use your nose.

However, if nasal breathing was restricting your ventilation greater than the typical 20%, Professor Dallam observed a negative impact on performance. He explained that you wouldn't be breathing enough air to oxygenate your blood and muscles sufficiently. Professor Dallam has been studying nasal versus oral breathing in labs, and although not all the data has been published yet, he notes that some people who aren't yet adapted are unable to ventilate sufficiently when only using the nose, resulting in higher lactate levels, reduced muscle oxygenation and a higher RPE.

He went on to compare subjects who struggled with nasal breathing during exercises with those who didn't, noting that those who had significant air hunger struggled when work intensity increase. In contrast, those who could manage the air hunger saw efficiency markers improve: lower ventilation, slightly reduced VO_2, stable lactate levels and air hunger with decreased RPE. The implication being that, 'There is a threshold for everyone, which, when reached, causes hypoventilation [under-breathing] until they adapt,' explained Professor Dallam.

Essentially everyone has a different starting point and a different threshold to nasal breathing. A 2009 study found that nasal breathing was possible up to 85% VO_2 max during running when some training and familiarisation had taken place.[6] A 2017 study had similar results, with nasal breathing possible up to around 80% of VO_2 max in non-adapted subjects.[7] Despite the subjects not being adapted, the researchers did highlight that up until their switch point, nasal breathing was more efficient. This seems pretty high, higher than you might expect. But what does that actually feel like and what sort of pace would that be? I wanted to find out for myself rather than just read about the research.

I organised my own VO_2 max test at Salford University in 2024 to put myself to the test. During the test there were three key 'switching points' for my breathing that I asked Dr Anna Robins to note down during the test. The final one was when I couldn't manage nasal breathing anymore and switched to my mouth. Very interestingly, it was exactly the point my body switched from aerobic to anaerobic energy systems – my second ventilatory threshold. That point was at 87.5% of my VO_2 max (55.0ml/kg/min), and I felt like I was working pretty hard by this point. I was running at 15km/hr with a 1% gradient, equivalent to 20min 5km pace, pretty close to my 5km PB.

It was an interesting experiment for me. I'd never done a VO_2 max test before. I can't lie and tell you that I wasn't happy about achieving a switch point beyond the quoted 80–85% in the literature. I'd done lots of work on my breathing and I wanted it to pay off. I knew my running performance had improved dramatically. It felt better, more controlled and more relaxed. Achieving 87.5% of VO_2 max before switching, which coincided with my ventilatory threshold, was quite an achievement. Dr Robins explained that the ventilatory threshold is when 'you can't supply oxygen quick enough and so switch from predominately aerobic to anaerobic and we see a steep climb in your lactate levels at that point'. Interestingly, despite all the fancy testing equipment that could calculate it, it took blood samples, thousands of pounds' worth of equipment and about a week until I got my results. Yet my breathing knew. My breathing told me when I'd hit my ventilatory threshold and switched from aerobic to anaerobic through immediate feedback, when I switched from using my nose to my mouth.

So maybe we can do more than we think with our nose? It also appears that practice makes a difference to whether someone is adapted or not.

Studies have found considerable variations in the switch point between individuals, and interestingly, the RPE for breathing rather than the amount of ventilation was more closely related to the switch point.[8] If the switch point is more subjective than a fixed ventilation level – and more closely linked to RPE, which we've seen can be affected by the way we breathe – surely this switching point and the intensity I can achieve with the benefits of nasal breathing are trainable? What's the difference with people who've trained it and are adapted to nasal breathing that Professor Dallam spoke of?

Training adaptations

According to Professor Dallam, adaptations from specifically training nasal breathing during running are both biochemical (tolerance to carbon dioxide) and mechanical (the amount of air you can move through your nose with your diaphragm). We become adapted to carbon dioxide if the levels are regularly increased, the receptors don't react as much and their response is down-regulated, 'the air hunger goes away,' he explained. By practising nasal breathing you get to increase your tolerance of carbon dioxide, as it's not leaving as quickly via the nose. A higher tolerance to carbon dioxide allows for superior breath control, meaning slower and more efficient breathing. He's not the only one to highlight the benefits. Research from 2020 in the *Journal of Sports Research* looked at both adapted subjects that had trained nasal breathing as well as those that had not.[9] The researchers concluded that 'the evidence suggests that exclusively nasal breathing is feasible for most people at moderate levels of aerobic exercise without specific adaptation, and that this breathing approach may also be achieved during heavy and maximal levels of aerobic exercise following a sustained period of use. Benefits of nasal breathing include a reduction in exercise-induced bronchoconstriction, improved ventilatory efficiency, and lower physiological economy for a given level of work.' This means nasal breathing is not just possible at moderate intensity for most people but it's also 'trainable'. When you practise it, you get better at it, the body seems to adapt positively, and you can do it at faster-paced running.

Professor Dallam also points out that nasal breathing can also help improve the mechanics of our breathing via diaphragmatic function. Adaptation over time means the diaphragm gets stronger, due to the increased resistance of the nose, and you use it more efficiently. The subsequent increase in ventilation at high work intensities increases tidal volume, meaning we can transfer oxygen more efficiently at the lungs and reduce sensations of air hunger.

Would the result be the same if I just do slow, deep breathing with my mouth? I'd still benefit from improving alveolar ventilation, presumably. Slow mouth breathing has been compared with slow nasal breathing in one study, and the mouth improved ventilatory efficiency when used slowly, but subjects still inhaled more air compared with nasal breathing, suggesting that other mechanisms are involved. In his book, Professor Dallam notes that this suggests 'other mechanisms that come into play during nasal breathing, such as improved diffusion resulting from improved ventilation to perfusion matching and/or greater production of nitric oxide, are not fully exploited when we simply try to slow our breathing frequency while breathing orally during exercise.'[10]

I saw this in my VO_2 max testing data. Just before I switched from nose to mouth, I was ventilating 79.5L/min and used 3.95L/min of oxygen (VO_2). My ventilatory efficiency ratio for oxygen was 79.5 / 3.95 = 20.13 (the lower the ratio, the more efficient you are). Once I switched to mouth breathing, I headed towards my VO_2 max and peaked at a total ventilation of 120.6L/min, and my VO_2 was 4.51L/min, so my ventilatory efficiency was 26.74 (120.6 / 4.51). It's still a relatively low ratio, meaning I was being efficient (30 is considered elite), but it wasn't as efficient as my nose. However, I was able to ventilate 50% more air in total (per minute) with my mouth and increase my total oxygen uptake by 14%, which allowed me to continue running gradually faster and faster for three more minutes after my switch point.

The good news for those of us who find nasal breathing difficult is that there are things we can learn from the benefits of nasal breathing that we can apply to mouth breathing, and there are intensities where mouth breathing is required. But it gets better still, training nasal breathing can actually help improve mouth breathing in runners, according to Professor Dallam. Research indicates that training nasal breathing improves ventilation efficiency even when you switch to mouth breathing. But it's not yet known if nasal breathing improves nasal efficiency, because it is superior from the start. Professor Dallam noted that a 2024 study at Baylor University found that four weeks of nasal breathing for 30 minutes at 70% of maximum heart rate resulted in a 29% increase in oxygen uptake and 19% when VO_2 max was retested at 85% and 100%, respectively, with mouth breathing.[11]

So, if you can do some of your training nasally the research suggests it even improves your mouth-breathing efficiency when you switch beyond your nasal threshold. Practising nasal breathing earns you the right to mouth breathe efficiently when you need it.

However, it's not just about efficiency and performance improvements. Those of us more interested in health and longevity will be keen to take up nasal breathing during running when they hear about the important protective nature of the nose for your heart.

Something clearly close to Professor Dallam's heart is the effect nasal breathing might have on it. He spoke passionately with a sense of hope that others would adopt it because, remember, he's not just a researcher, he's also an endurance athlete; he's seen friends suffer with heart problems that he's noticed could be linked to how we breathe in endurance sports.

Professor Dallam explained that we are seeing a higher degree of fibrosis in endurance athletes, with increased incidence of myocardial scarring and atrial fibrillation, which he and other researchers believe may be linked to the way we breathe during exercise. He explained, 'Because we breathe too hard and too fast orally during intense exercise, creating relative hyperventilation, reducing carbon dioxide and the dilation can't happen and the heart can't pump.' He's co-authored a literature review and theoretical analysis with respiratory scientist Martin McPhilimey, who explained that because nasal breathing helps slow the breathing rate, it helps reduce stress on the heart by reducing overall sympathetic tone and reducing arousal. 'When we reduce the load on the heart, we have less chance of arrhythmias,' he explained. They also suggest the increase in carbon dioxide in the blood from nasal breathing helps improve blood flow through vasodilation at the heart, essentially meaning the heart doesn't have to work as hard compared with fast mouth breathing which increases stress and the cardiovascular workload.

At the end of our fascinating interview, Professor Dallam left us with these encouraging words: 'exercise is good for you, but if you breathed better during exercise, it's even better for you!'

Start slow and get used to the nose

As we've seen, there are two elements we need to train to adopt nasal breathing and experience the benefits in some of our training: carbon dioxide tolerance and the strength of our diaphragm. Luckily for us, the resistance the nose provides compared with the mouth ensures a stimulus in training to improve both.

Patrick McKeown explains that air hunger is stronger at the start but diminishes as your body becomes used to increased carbon dioxide levels when nasal breathing during exercise. He noted when studying athletes: 'I found that elite athletes have a lower chemosensitivity to carbon dioxide, regardless of whether they trained breathing specifically.' So good news for those who are fitter: the more trained and conditioned you are, the easier you'll potentially find getting used to nasal breathing for some of your training.

Professor Dallam suggests finding a running pace below your nasal threshold (NT) that is comfortable, and gradually increase the pace (which you learn how to measure in the assessments in chapter 7). Over time, by adapting to the increase in carbon dioxide you'll experience and by getting used to the added resistance to airflow the diaphragm will have to overcome, nasal breathing becomes easier and your diaphragm gets stronger.

You can't change the shape and size of your nose (but I have a few tools in the next chapter to help your nose breathing specifically);

however, everything else is trainable. You can improve carbon dioxide sensitivity and your psychological relationship with feeling out of breath. You can strengthen your diaphragm and develop better biomechanical breathing patterns and habits that all make nasal breathing easier and breathing in general more efficient. As Patrick said encouragingly at the end of our interview, 'You just need to practise.'

> **TRY THIS**
>
> 1. Perform some of your training runs breathing nasally. You choose how much, but start with your slower-paced runs initially – warm-ups are a good time to practise nasal breathing too, if you do one!
> 2. Choose a running pace that is manageable and the air hunger is not too uncomfortable.
> 3. Be patient – it doesn't instantly feel like a 'magic bullet' – the magic bullet is always consistency in training.

We all make mistakes but don't make mine!

It's not always as simple as just shutting your mouth, and my personal experience highlights the mistakes I don't want you to make. I mentioned at the start of the chapter sucking air up my nose like a vacuum cleaner. I was doing nasal breathing at all costs regardless of the pace I was running. I was trying to force adaptation with my nose rather than allowing it to happen, and I had no idea of my nasal threshold. It wasn't comfortable and, to be honest, I'm surprised I didn't give up. I think the saving grace was the motivation that I was initially doing it to help with my brain health after recovering from my traumatic brain injury. It made it more important to stick with it. Don't make the mistake of trying to force it, or you might give up on it too early before the adaptations have time to do their magic.

The other big mistake I made was assuming nasal breathing meant I was diaphragmatically breathing efficiently. It's true the nose provides more resistance that, for some people helps recruit the diaphragm, but not for all of us initially. If you have developed strong accessory breathing muscles because the brain likes the path of least resistance, when resistance increases with nasal breathing, the habit of lifting the upper chest can be activated more strongly. The fact I forced my nasal breathing too much on runs, and made it very stressful for myself, will be one of the reasons I was still stuck in upper chest-dominant breathing patterns. A weak diaphragm, a tight ribcage and a learned compensatory breathing pattern also contributed. We often need more than just shutting the biggest hole in your face. The good news for you is that my struggles have meant I've developed specific breathing techniques you can adapt in your training. You'll get help with your breathing mechanics and diaphragm in chapter 8, breathing mobilisations to open up your tight ribcage in chapter 9, plus all the other practical tips that lie ahead in the chapters to come.

You might even be surprised at how quickly it can change, like at a workshop I ran in Scotland with everyday runners and gym users of all ages and abilities. In just one session, once we'd worked on optimising their airway, activating their diaphragm and had some practice in getting used to the sensation of how it feels to use their nose while exercising, it felt better and easier. When I asked the group to put their hand up at the end of the session if they achieved a higher intensity with their nose than what they managed at the start and if it surprised them, everyone – from the 18-year-old just starting to the retired pensioner, even the weekend warrior and everyone in between – put their hand up. They'd improved their threshold in just one session.

I said we'd look at the science of what's possible with our nose and why it might be beneficial to use some nasal breathing during our running sessions. I promised we wouldn't get our knickers in a twist and hopefully yours aren't, as you're encouraged by the science you've learned. Further encouragement is that I've seen time and time again with athletes that we can do more with our nose than we might initially think; we can train to improve our capacity and benefit from the efficiency of nasal breathing.

Those who've been paying close attention might have noticed an interesting link between what Professor Dallam has seen is possible with nasal breathing and what Professor Dempsey believed the lung was capable of. Have you made the link? Both appear to have a limit around 85% VO_2 max. Interesting, right? Could it be that we aren't designed to run at higher intensities than 85% of VO_2 max, not just because the nose struggles with it but because the lungs also struggle? Could this be the reason why above this intensity our auto setting becomes seemingly counterproductive and less efficient as we naturally start panting with the mouth, the upper chest bouncing up and down and restricting our tidal volume? Our breathing wants us to stop if we allow the auto to take over. Or if we haven't trained our auto at those higher thresholds. With training though, nasal breathing could be your 'secret to improved health and athletic performance and recovery' as described in an article published by EC Pulmonology and Respiratory Medicine.[12]

Clearly not all elite athletes and runners are nasal breathing all of the time. As we've seen, it depends on the individual and the intensity of running, and the closer to 85% VO_2 max, the less beneficial it might be. Yet we've seen it is possible to improve your mouth breathing when you are pushing your limits by using nasal breathing in some of your training. I call it 'earning the right to mouth breathe'. Rather than letting mouth breathing be a compensatory pattern, let's get better and learn from the efficiency of the nose, by better controlling our breathing rate and utilising the diaphragm.

If you do your homework like the runner in a study from 2019 – who changed all training to nasal breathing for six weeks and improved his mouth breathing 5km time by 6% – you'll be sowing seeds of adaptation with nasal breathing in training and reaping the benefits when using your mouth in a race or training at higher intensities.[13]

The choice is yours, but the benefits are for us all.

For now, keep your mouth closed as you continue reading, create nasal breathing as a habit away from your training and benefit from its protective qualities: fewer upper respiratory tract illnesses, less sympathetic activation, as well as protecting your heart. You only get one of those, and you want to look after it!

Next, we're going to learn about the importance of the airway behind the holes in your face, and what some experts consider to be the most important muscle in your body. Like me, you might be very surprised not just by what muscle it is but the effect it can have on your breathing while running.

Key takeaways

- Research into nasal breathing has been limited because of restrictions with testing procedures.
- Nasal breathing improves ventilatory efficiency, meaning more oxygen is extracted at the lungs per breath.
- The resistance of nasal breathing naturally slows the respiratory rate. As long as it's not restricting your total ventilation too much, you can oxygenate efficiently while breathing more slowly and calmly.
- When you adapt to nasal breathing, you can see improvements in lower ventilation, lower lactate and reduced perception of effort up to around 80–85% of VO_2 max.
- Training nasally helps you 'earn the right to mouth breathe' more efficiently when you are running at higher intensities, as it trains your diaphragm and your carbon dioxide tolerance.
- Create nasal breathing as a good habit in your day-to-day life when not training: by shutting the big hole in your face when you're not running!

> Breathing is the most fundamental thing we have to do, and when we are running you are only going to do more of it, it's crazy we've never considered training it.
>
> **Dr Martin Yelling**

CHAPTER 6

Shut your mouth, lose your ego and train your airway

You're about to learn about the surprising structure of your airway from a dentist, why it's often a missing piece of our breathing puzzle and meet the most underrated but most important muscle in the human body. We'll finish with some hacks to help keep your nose open and the air flowing freely, making nasal breathing more comfortable on easy runs.

It started with a snotty affair

I love a jigsaw puzzle. I got a 1000-piece Snowdonia OS map for my 41st birthday from my mum. Like any jigsaw puzzle it's a complete mess at the start. It makes no sense at all and starting is the hardest bit. Getting the first few pieces in place is the most important but also the hardest part as you start. You look for the edge pieces first because they have some straight lines you can recognise and form the foundation of the puzzle, the outline. Once they are in place, you sort of get an idea of what you're working with. The picture gets a bit clearer; other pieces of the puzzle start to fit into place and it gets easier. Despite the gaps being completely blank, it starts to make sense and you make faster progress filling those blanks as you go.

It's similar getting started with training breathing and running. You need to know what the pieces of the puzzle are, where to start and which are the outline pieces to put down first to form a foundation. This chapter is exactly that. It's the start, but remember, just the start. It forms the foundation upon which you'll be able to build and put more pieces of your puzzle together. Everyone's starting point is a little different and mine was certainly a messy one.

I close my mouth, tell myself, *This is better for you* and try to convince myself nasal breathing will solve all my problems. I set off down the road from my house, thinking I'd head to the park and do my usual 5km route. I got 50m down the road, started sucking air up my nose and I felt like I was suffocating slightly. I've not got particularly big nostrils and they started closing in as I sucked air in faster and I started to panic. I tried to remind myself about the benefits of nasal breathing I'd been reading about in the research. The feeling of suffocation as my nostrils struggled to supply my brain with a sense of enough air and oxygen was unpleasant. I tried to convince myself, *Its ok, it's just carbon dioxide not leaving as quickly*. It almost feels like you're drowning. As snot started to pour out of my nose into my mouth, it literally happened. I couldn't handle it any longer. I stopped running, took a sigh of relief (which basically dumped off carbon dioxide that was accumulating in my lungs and blood at a higher rate than my receptors were used to). I wiped the snot from my nose and mouth. Feeling dejected, I managed about 150m, which got me to the end of my road. Not exactly the 5km nasal run I'd envisioned.

Wow, this is hard. If nasal breathing is supposed to be better for me and better for my running, why does it feel impossible to me? I thought. I reminded myself of the brain injury I'd sustained about six years previously. The reason I was trying to improve my breathing, which the brain injury had put out of whack, was much bigger than getting better at running. It was about getting better at breathing and using running as a tool to help me experience my breathing and increase my awareness of it. That was a key turning point for me. A realisation that I was terrible at breathing. It wasn't going under the radar any longer. My nose as a 'use it or lose it' organ had lost it.

I had some serious work to do, but because initially it wasn't about being good or better at running, that allowed my ego to relax and let me run or jog as slowly as necessary to manage the airflow through my nose. It's not that we have to do all of our running breathing nasally – as we've seen from the research, most people need to use their mouth more than their nose at around 85% VO_2 max. But I was jogging, it wasn't even a warm-up pace, and I couldn't do it breathing nasally.

It was time to get to work. Work that would be life-changing for me and, longer term, transform my running ability. It would ignite a love of ultra-running, eventually allowing me to push my limits far beyond what I ever imagined possible.

My small airway has taught me many lessons

The more I've tried to improve my own breathing through experimentation and the more I've helped runners and athletes of all sports improve theirs, it's become very clear that we need to 'line up all our ducks' when it comes to breathing to transform our running. Lining up those ducks is about optimising all the components of breathing that are trainable and in your control. Certain things are less in your control. For example, a thin face restricts the size of your airway, or you might have a tongue that's too big for your mouth – or is your mouth too small for your tongue and teeth? These things that are part of your DNA dictate how easily the air can come in and out of your nose and how easily it will pass through your airway. Your tongue, you'll learn later, is key not just to your airway but also your mechanics, as it's connected to your diaphragm through lines of fascia. Fascia is the fascinating link between all your muscles and connective tissue (ligaments and tendons). There are specific lines of fascia that pioneering researcher Thomas Myers, author of *Anatomy Trains*, has identified: The deep front line is the one which connects the tongue with the diaphragm and travels all the way down to your big toe. It essentially means that your tongue and airway muscles will influence your diaphragm; hence the importance of your tongue as a muscle on your breathing.

During my journey I've had to try to optimise my less-than-ideal DNA. Although I'd probably love to have a nose, nostrils and airway like David Rudisha, I'm grateful in a way for my narrow face and poor airway structure (my high palate) because it's meant nasal breathing has been a difficult journey for me. That difficult journey has led me to dive deeper and explore every nook and cranny of the airway to see how we can optimise it. Without my struggles I wouldn't have been forced to look at breathing and the airway with the detail I have. I wouldn't have been able to write this book authentically, especially this important chapter. It's led me down some unexpected interesting avenues, such as the dentist who taught me tongue exercises to improve my airway and breathing, which was when I went from a snotty mess to a relaxed, smiling nasal-breathing runner. A lesson for me that started with the biggest turning point in my life.

Importance of your upper airway

'We were all about to laugh, as it was funny the way you and Phil were trying to catch the same pass, you hit the deck like a bag of potatoes,' explained Shawsy. 'But when you hit the floor you started having a fit and I helped put you in the recovery position, made sure you didn't swallow your tongue and we shouted the physio over.' As Shawsy relived the brain injury that ended my rugby career, luckily my memory of the weeks surrounding that day has never come back. I'm glad, as I wouldn't want to remember them.

I'd become so susceptible to being knocked out (through repeated concussions over my 13-year professional rugby career) that an innocuous collision with a teammate, playing touch in a warm-up, left me having a seizure on the field. Luckily for me, Shawsy remembered some first aid training and the importance of my not swallowing my tongue.

We knew nothing about breathing, but anyone who's been on an emergency first aid course will remember the final part of the 'recovery position' is to tilt the head to open the airway. When there is a possibility of you swallowing your tongue and potentially dying, we take breathing and our airway alignment far more seriously than in day-to-day life or running.

Breathing in day-to-day life is still obviously important but we never tend to think about opening our airway by lifting the chin. When we are running, our breathing and airway are even more important, as breathing volume and rate are challenged by physical exercise. Yet we still have no understanding of the importance of the airway. Your airway isn't your nose or your mouth. They are just the holes in your face, the gateway to the airway, two different routes into the same place. Air needs to go back and down to your lungs.

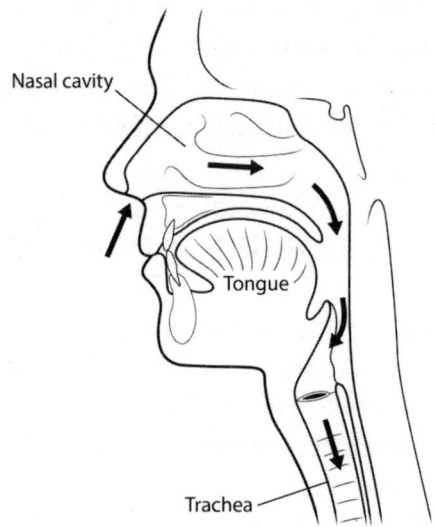

You probably thought you were supposed to breathe *up* your nose!

The most important muscle in your body

The importance of the airway was unexpectedly pointed out to me at the dentist and has since transformed my breathing and sleep (like all muscles, the muscles of the airway relax when you sleep, so has a huge impact on your sleep quality). I thought I was going to have my teeth checked when my wife booked us into a new 'biological dentist', but to my surprise it wasn't until about 45 minutes into the appointment we even discussed my teeth! When I walked into the Wonder of Wellness clinic little did I know I was about to be introduced to one of the most important and overlooked muscles in the human body: the tongue.

As strange as it might seem, the thing in your mouth with all of your beautiful taste buds on, that wiggles around when you speak to make difference noises is actually a muscle. A unique muscle, as it's the only muscle attached at just one end. It has an important role in our ability to taste and communicate, but its most important job is what's overlooked. How it affects your breathing and particularly its role in supporting your jaw and airway and its connection to your diaphragm. I had no idea about any of this as I went into my first appointment.

When I sat down in the dentist chair with Annie, a dental and myofunctional therapist, it was just like any other dentist chair, but the assessment to follow was like no other. It started not with my teeth but with my tongue and my airway, 'because how you breathe has a huge impact on your dental hygiene,' Annie explained. I liked the sound of this, someone else geek-ing out on breathing but from a whole different angle that I'd not explored. That appointment lasted about 30 minutes longer than the allotted time because I had so many questions. Not wanting to hold things up any further, I organised two interviews with Annie and the co-founder of the practice, Dr Sebastian Lomas, a biological dentist. I wanted to know what we can learn from biological dentistry and myofunctional therapy to improve our breathing for running.

Where should your tongue live?

Something Annie had pointed out in my assessment were the marks on the sides of my tongue that confirmed what I suspected, my tongue was too big for my mouth. But that wasn't strictly correct, as she explained, 'Your mouth is too small for your tongue, hence the marks on the tongue, and importantly your mouth dictates the size of your airway. Especially the top jaw and palate.' For 50% of Dr Lomas's patients, it's the same. He explained factors such as genetics, health issues or tooth extraction can all result in a smaller mouth and not enough room for the tongue, meaning it sits further back and blocks the airway.

According to Dr Lomas, the tongue is one of the most important muscles in the human body because of its direct relationship with breathing. I was interested to know if training our tongue and improving the 'openness' of the airway would help nasal breathing during exercise and running. Could we improve how much and how easily air can travel through our nose and airway? 'Efficiency of breathing is to do with resistance of air and pressure of how its inhaled,' explained Dr Lomas. Where your tongue is and how it's placed in the mouth affects this. 'With tongue position suctioned to the soft palate there is less turbulence of airflow, less resistance and therefore in terms of airflow, breathing is more efficient. When the tongue is not sealed to the roof of the mouth the air coming in "spins" and you get more turbulence at the back of your mouth, creating more resistance.'

Could less turbulence and resistance to airflow keep our nostrils from closing in on themselves when we feel like we're sucking air in when running faster? Dr Lomas explained that it can affect the nostrils. 'Try breathing in fast through your nose with your tongue loose at the bottom of your jaw and notice how your nostrils collapse in on themselves due to the turbulence of the airflow. Now try it with your tongue suctioned to the roof of your mouth and notice the difference.' Wow, sure enough, Dr Lomas was right. My tongue changed my breathing instantly.

The nostrils closing in on themselves during running with nasal breathing is something that I'd experienced any time I tried to run at a decent pace. My poor tongue posture and its lack of muscle tone was having a negative effect on my ability to nasal breathe during running.

Dr Lomas explained, 'Your tongue position will not only transform your breathing by supporting your airway and jaw, but it even affects your breathing mechanics as the tongue is connected through fascia within the deep front line to your diaphragm.' I wondered if the tongue position is important when we start running or if it's just important for our everyday life. 'At the start it will be harder when running and you'll need to be more conscious of it. It won't feel "normal" but that's normal when doing something new or different,' explained Dr Lomas. He added that it's really important when running with nasal breathing, because as your diaphragm is pulling down (you'll learn more about this in chapter 8), it will become harder to keep your tongue up as your diaphragm pulls on that deep front line of fascia all the way up to your tongue. It pulls against the tongue position you're trying to reach at the top of the palate. It appears that tongue strength in that position is even more critical during exercise than during rest.

As already discussed, there are times when you'll likely be required to use the bigger hole in your face when running at higher intensities. When mouth breathing, the tongue must be down or you won't be able to breathe through your mouth. If your airway lacks muscle tone, when your tongue is down during mouth breathing, you're more susceptible to airway restriction. The link through fascia the tongue has with the diaphragm may also be a reason why mouth breathing is linked to upper chest breathing and less activation of the diaphragm.

I'd learned the airway is one of the most important things affecting our breathing. The alignment of your neck, jaw and tongue position all affect the openness of your airway and therefore how easily air will flow. Your airway is about the same circumference as your thumb. Just a centimetre or two. If the head is forward and out of alignment, this compromises the airway, compressing the space the air needs to flow down and squashing the 1–2cm space from the back of the neck. If the chin is tucked and pulled back – a posture many athletes adopt having been told a 'tucked chin' is good posture – you compromise the space for your 1–2cm airway by pulling the jaw back and ramming it into that space, which is supposed to be allowing air to flow.

During running you need that airway to be open and supported to manage the velocity and volume of air coming in, and your tongue is integral to this. When you can manage the airflow through the smaller holes in your face, it's also easier to stay relaxed. The correct tongue position not only helps the airflow and supports the jaw and airway, but research has linked the tongue to the parasympathetic nervous system.[1] Greater parasympathetic and reduced sympathetic activity when the tongue is on the roof of the mouth can help us runners stay more relaxed.

Finally, it's not just breathing the tongue affects. In a 2014 study when the tongue was at the roof of the mouth compared with a mid-position, subjects increased knee flexion strength by 30%.[2] Stronger knees just from having the tongue on the roof of the mouth, that sounds crazy. Maybe

Dr Lomas is right – the tongue is the most important muscle in the body. What other muscle has that much influence over other body parts?

He finished with a strong claim: 'Training your airway is the best-kept secret in sport.' But most people don't know why they need to do it, let alone how to train it. He and Annie recommend simple exercises to perform, which I was keen to learn because changing the shape and size of my jaw, palate and skull seemed like a much more difficult job! Narrowly missing out on the Olympic boxing team for the London 2012 Olympics shifted Dr Lomas's focus to becoming a dentist. What I appreciated was that he understood the importance of breathing from a physical exercise perspective, despite his focus as a dentist on oral and overall health. He's lived and breathed life as an athlete and was generous with sharing this new knowledge with me on the airway and tongue. I was thirsty, and he was filling my cup!

Exercise: Tongue training and how to keep your nostrils open

Annie explained that tongue exercises improve the muscle tone in your tongue and airway and can show where the tongue should live in the roof of your mouth. So, what is the correct position for the tongue, how do you put it there and am I doing it right? I hear you say (because they were the same first questions I asked).

'Most people can put tip of the tongue up, just behind back of the teeth, but that still leaves the important parts of the tongue, the middle and especially the back of the tongue, away from the soft palate which will contribute to unnecessary turbulence to airflow that will only get worse when running,' explained Dr Lomas. He has two exercises for us that double up as a way of checking positioning, as well as exercises for good tongue posture and tongue 'toning' – I bet you never thought you'd be training your tongue when you picked up a book about breathing for runners – neither did I!

These two exercises are great as a 'test' to check tongue position, tightness and strength, but they are also key exercises that Dr Lomas uses with his clients to teach the correct position and get strong at having it 'live in the correct place' at the roof of your mouth.

EXERCISE: TRAIN YOUR TONGUE AND AIRWAY

1. **Tongue clicks**
   - Have your mouth slightly open.
   - Lift the tongue to the roof of the mouth and try to make a 'clicking' noise as the tongue pings off the roof of the palate.
   - If you're making a clicking sound, that's it. Simples!
   - Notice where the tongue is sitting just before it 'clicks' off the roof of the mouth. That's where your tongue is meant to live. It's like all that space between your teeth in the roof of your mouth is its home.
   - Finally, I want you to appreciate the suction you create to set up the position to make the clicking sound. You'll use that suction in the second exercise.

2. **Suction and stretch**
   - Perform another 'tongue click' but this time rather than letting the tongue ping off and make a 'clicking' sound, I want you to do it in slow motion, so slowly that you create more suction so it stays there.
   - Keep the tongue there by progressively creating more and more suction as you open your mouth gradually wider.
   - Open your mouth as wide as you can until you feel like your tongue is about to 'ping' off, but keep it there.
   - You'll feel the bottom of the tongue stretching (especially if it's tight).
   - You'll also feel the tongue working hard to create a strong suction to keep it there.
   - This is both strengthening the suction ability of the tongue as well as stretching the tightness that builds up at the base of it.

Dr Lomas likes to have patients build up to being able to perform this 'suction and stretch' exercise for three minutes. Set a timer, then each time it pings off, after 5–10 seconds of rest, go again, and try to accumulate three minutes of the exercise.

A nice simple way to check that you've sealed the tongue to the roof of the mouth correctly is to keep your mouth open, pinch your nose and try to breathe in through your mouth. If the tongue is fully sealed to the roof of your mouth, it will be blocking your mouth's route to the airway – you won't be able to breathe through the mouth if the tongue is correctly sealed. It's a nice added benefit of correct tongue posture. If the tongue is sealed and living in the correct place, it encourages natural nasal breathing at rest.

'How much suction does it need?' I asked. 'In general life, to have it in the correct position, just a light suction so that the tongue holds itself up with the suction so you're not having to "push it up there",' explained Dr Lomas. But when training the tongue with the suction exercise, he suggests, you should push it up to train the strength of your tongue maximally to develop that strength and improve muscle tone.

A nice progression once you can perform the exercise for three minutes is to introduce a head tilt so that the head is tilted back while performing the suction and stretch, as this position targets toning the airway tube at the same time.

If these exercises are not possible due to a tongue tie, I suggest reaching out to a health practitioner, like Dr Lomas, as tongue tie can be released by a small procedure.

Within a number of weeks and certainly within two months, Dr Lomas says you should feel improvements in your airway and how your breathing feels. If that feels too long for those of you with little patience, I've seen improvements with athletes I'm coaching within just one training session. By focusing on the correct tongue position and activating the suction correctly with this exercise – the athletes and I have been amazed.

Your nose is just the tip of the iceberg

Around the same time as learning about the airway, I had a strange and scary, yet enlightening experience about the airway, which really brings it to life. All the master trainers with the Oxygen Advantage were at Patrick McKeown's training centre on the west coast of Ireland in Galway. We had a number of CPD (continuing professional development) sessions and one quite literally blew my mind.

Brian Marabella handed out a Q-tip (cotton bud) to everyone (please don't try this at home). We had to dip the cotton bud in some essential oils, and I wondered where he was going to put it as he explained how this would help clear our noses and airway. As Brian demonstrated and encouraged us to do the same, I couldn't believe my eyes when this Q-tip seemingly disappeared into his face! 'Where the hell did that just go, Brian?' I shouted!

As weird as it seemed, I wanted to try it for myself. *Where did it go?* I followed Brian's instructions, starting to slowly push the Q-tip horizontally backwards into one of the three canals that Brian explained go backwards, not up the nose. As weird as it felt at first, this Q-tip started disappearing into my face. It was ridiculous but amazing all at the start time. My mind flashed back to the conversations with Annie and interview with Dr Lomas. *It's going in the airway they were describing.* The nose is just the tip of the iceberg – it's not the important thing, the airway is. It goes right back into your face! Of course, it does, it goes back to your throat and then down to your lungs.

Why are we all trying to breathe up our nose? I thought to myself, *the air needs to go backwards*. With that thought and my tongue in the correct position, I took a breath in and again my breathing was transformed. I was breathing 'back' rather than 'up' my nose, my tongue was supporting my airway and jaw, and the airflow felt glorious. Breathing felt very easy. Effortless.

The Q-tip uncovered what we can't see. It showed the airway in a different light. Where it actually is, the direction of the canals and how far back it goes. I gained a new dimension to my understanding of the airway, and everything Dr Lomas and Annie said made more sense. It was like I could see and imagine the airway properly. The Q-tip demonstration is something I've used time and time again as a demonstration to both shock and inform people when I'm teaching about the airway. It always raises a few eyebrows, as well as transforming how people breathe. Like Claire Woodfield, a beginner runner in Scotland who said, 'Since the workshop I've started "breathing into my face" as you coached us, and I can't tell you the difference it's made to my breath control. I even feel like I can run longer already!'

> **TRY THIS**

Try breathing up the nose compared with breathing 'into the face' or back:

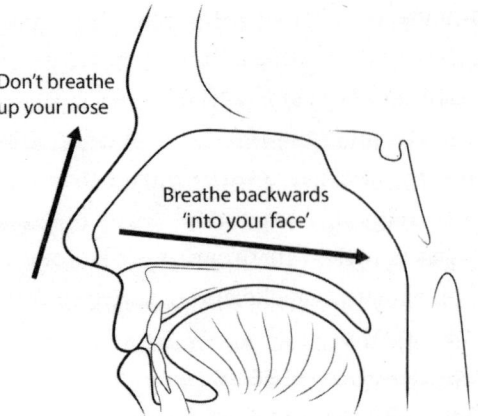

Breathing back is the simplest but biggest game changer for your breathing!

Feel the difference for yourself:

- Place one hand on your chest and the other hand on your abdomen so you can feel the changes in the mechanics of where you breathe.
- Firstly, try breathing up your nose, with the tongue at the bottom of your mouth; notice the airflow and how you lift your ribcage and upper chest up vertically.
- Now optimise the alignment of your neck and airway by looking slightly up so that you lift your chin only a small amount, about an inch, to help open the airway. You should feel like your palate is stacked on top of your throat.
- Have the mouth softly closed, jaw relaxed with teeth not touching and place as much of your tongue to the roof of your mouth as you can (front, middle and even back of the tongue).
- Create some light suction to keep the tongue there.
- Now breathe 'into the face' through the nose, rather than up the nose.
- Follow the airflow to the back of the throat.
- Compare it with how it felt breathing up your nose – which hand moves more now?

How easy does the airflow feel? Breathing should feel more effortless. You should also notice your lower ribcage expand, as this helps activate the diaphragm, compared with the upper chest lifting when you breathed up your nose.

On your next easy run, think about having your tongue up and breathe back, breathing into your face through your nose rather than up it. One of the most important bits of advice I can give you starting out with nasal running is to make sure you are running at a pace slow enough that you can relax and practise these two things. Don't go at a pace that feels stressful with your breathing. Let your nose dictate the pace of your run. Give it a few weeks and that pace will improve.

Two nose tricks up your sleeve

To help the sensation of airflow in the nostrils, it can be helpful to have a few tricks up your sleeve to help keep them open. I've got two simple yet game-changing nasal hacks for you. Both are free, they don't require you to put anything on your nose or up your nose, such as nasal strips or nasal dilators (although they can be a good option for some people). I like to keep things as simple as possible, plus both of these are a bit fun too!

Option 1: Increase nasal ventilation by over 25% with turtle power

The first option is something I developed organically to help my nostrils stay open when the faster airflow was causing them to collapse in on themselves when I ran faster, which I call 'turtle power'! This works an absolute treat in the short term. Interestingly it was my second switch point that I mentioned in the last chapter during my VO_2 max testing. This was the point I had to start using turtle power to meet the ventilation demand as the VO_2 max test ramped up, which turned out to be when lactate increased as I transitioned from heart rate zone 3 towards zone 4. Proof of its effectiveness was that before switching to turtle power, my nose was restricting me to around 63L/min, but when I switched to turtle power I was able to gradually increase it to 79.5L/min, a massive 26% increase in total ventilation with my nose.

I call it turtle power because you sort of position your mouth to make it look a bit like a turtle's mouth, plus I was a fan of Teenage Mutant Ninja Turtles as a kid, and this felt like a 'power up' moment.

> **TRY THIS**
>
> **How to turtle power**
> - First put your tongue in the correct position at the roof of the mouth.
> - Wrap your top lip around and over your top teeth. This creates some tension around the bottom of your nostrils, and sort of stretches them.
> - Bring your bottom lip up to meet your rolled-over top lip, forming the turtle-like mouth posture.

You might look a bit funny, but you won't care when you feel how amazing nasal breathing is like this. With your turtle power, breathe in as fast as you like and notice how your nostrils stay open and how much air and how quickly you can ventilate like this. You'll notice less restriction of airflow and no nostril collapse – you're welcome!

Option 2: Power of the smile – Vassos and Kipchoge

The other option is similar in mechanism but different in appearance. Vassos Alexander, runner, author and radio host, who converted all his running to nasal breathing, even his sub-3-hour marathon, told me something in our interview that he pinched off Kipchoge that helps his nostrils stay open. 'When I smile like Kipchoge, not only does it help me with stopping the nostrils closing in, it makes everyone I run past smile back at me.'

As we spoke it was very clear that Vassos was passionate not just about nasal breathing for his running performance but also the effect smiling had on his run as a whole and the people who saw him smiling while he ran through the parks of London. I wonder how much the power of the smile has on the 'feel-good factor', which may also play a part in helping us runners feel more relaxed. It's always nice when someone smiles at you. If you smile at someone else, it's nice for them too, it doesn't matter if you're just doing it to keep your nostrils open.

The wider the smile, the more stretch you'll put on the tissues, skin and cartilage of your nostrils to help them stay open. So bigger smiles will help with your nasal breathing; you could even go as far as to say, the faster you want to run with nasal breathing, the bigger your smile needs to be. Maybe that's why Kipchoge was beaming at the end of his sub-two-hour marathon world record?

We all have a different starting point

The starting point for each runner very much depends on their starting point. Some, like me, will find it extremely hard, maybe even a snot fest! Others will take to it straight away like it's the best thing they've ever done. Professional Ironman athlete Kerry Hickson was one of those. Having discussed some benefits of nasal breathing on 'easy' runs, Kerry decided to try nasal breathing on her next 10km tempo run.

She reported, 'It felt great. I felt less fatigued, recovered faster and the run itself felt easier.' If you're thinking that was just because the pace was slow, think again. Kerry's tempo runs are at a 4min/km pace, and this particular 10km was just under 40 minutes – that's not slow!

So not everyone finds it as difficult as I did at the start, and I've had countless messages from all sorts of runners who report benefits from the very first time they try it in easy runs or during cardio in the gym. In Kerry's case, she is clearly a fantastic athlete and extremely well-conditioned, and that conditioning will have played into the ease in which she was able to integrate nasal breathing into that type of running session.

One mistake I'd love to share with you, so you don't make the same one, is assuming it's a case of nasal breathing at all costs because you've read about so many benefits. I was so committed at the start I was determined to carry out nasal breathing regardless of the type of run or terrain. Desperately trying to nasal breathe while running up a steep hill when you've not yet adapted, without your tongue in the right position and your airway lacking tone because you've never trained it, is quite stressful. Your nose acts more like a vacuum than a normal set of nostrils, as you suck air inefficiently with poor breathing mechanics. Staying relaxed was the last thing on my mind; it was the opposite of relaxing, as I was trying not to drown or suffocate. I was uninformed, undertrained and not adapted. I'd made a start, but I was missing the point to a degree.

Once I'd swallowed my ego and dropped my pace to the point where I could breathe nasally, things finally started to improve. I started to piece more of the puzzle together and allowed for more time for adaptation, and I began to see some serious progress. Progress that started with running slower. Letting my nose dictate the pace of my run, rather than my Strava, training plan or ego. That's when things started to change.

Let the nose dictate the pace (not your ego) to get started

The best thing to do at the start is shut the big hole in your face, swallow your ego, put your tongue up, breathe back rather than up and let the nose dictate the pace of your running. No matter how slow that is initially, so you can stay relaxed. That is the simplest and best way to get started with the basics of improving your nasal breathing, especially if you are a beginner when it comes to running.

If you're patient, as you adapt, things start to feel easier, and not just your breathing but your running as a whole, which will be reflected in your heart rate. Initially I was just running a few kilometres at a time but managing around 6:30min/km pace, where my heart rate would normally be around 140bpm. I noticed with my more efficient breathing that my heart rate was down at 130bpm. Without trying to change my pace but just literally following my nose and letting it dictate the pace, I was adapting, and my body was finding running easier.

As the weeks and months passed, my running pace nasally started to increase. I was able to run 6:00min/km, then 5:30min/km and so on. My heart rate at a given pace now was around 10bpm slower than before. Nasal breathing wasn't just helping me regulate pace and keep me feeling calm and relaxed, it was actually making my cardiovascular system more efficient – my heart was working less to run at the same pace. This adaptation took a bit of time, but it wasn't a hack, it was a training adaptation of nasal breathing on my easy runs. It was the start of the improved efficiency that Professor Dallam spoke of.

This builds a foundation, a bit like an aerobic base but with nasal breathing. When you do faster-paced sessions, you want to have earned the right to mouth breathe rather than slipping into habitual compensatory breathing patterns. Nasal breathing at lower intensities helps train your breathing through the diaphragm and enable better breath control for when you have to mouth breathe. There is a whole chapter called 'When the nose isn't enough' so don't worry, there are plenty of tricks, tips and hacks waiting for you when you're ready to really open up the pace. But for now, be patient. The start is about building a base – a foundation and earning the right to mouth breathe.

A final reminder that in our day-to-day life of normal activities, it should be a non-negotiable to have your lips together, teeth not touching, jaw relaxed and breathing quietly through your nose (back, not up) in a relaxed fashion with your diaphragm. This creates a foundation of good breathing habits that you can build on when you start running.

We've been equipped with tools to train our tongue and improve our airway. You've got hacks like turtle power to increase nasal ventilation by potentially over 25%, as well as the power of the smile that Vassos stole from the beaming Kipchoge. When you can keep your nostrils open and the airway clear and supported, finding a pace that's comfortable to get started with becomes easier. As you begin to hone and benefit from the efficiency of nasal breathing, you'll be breathing less but oxygenating efficiently, bringing a sense of calm and control to your breathing and that all-important relaxation.

It's going to lay a foundation for you that as you adapt, you'll be able to run faster, longer and stronger with a lower heart rate. Practising nasal breathing during running even makes you better at mouth breathing when the running pace is beyond your nasal threshold – but you have to earn the right for that.

Key takeaways

- Your tongue is a crucial muscle for your airway and together they are a foundational piece of the nasal breathing puzzle.
- The tongue supports the jaw, and the neck position affects the openness of your airway, along with your tongue position.
- Your tongue should be gently suctioned to the roof of the mouth when nasal breathing, which reduces turbulence in the airway and makes the airflow easier.
- Open your airway by having the chin slightly up, the tongue in the roof of the mouth and breathe back rather than up the nose.
- Use turtle power or the power of the smile to give your nasal ventilation a potential 26% boost by keeping the nostrils open in faster-paced runs.

I've been running for fitness on and off since I was about 11 years old, and even back then, I remember breath being the first thing to go – the thing that would stop me in my tracks.

Years later, learning from Jacko completely changed my relationship with running, and with myself. 'Keeping it nasal' has truly changed my life. Not only has nasal breathing transformed my endurance and recovery, but learning the power of down-regulation, especially after runs or during times of high stress, has brought a deeper calm into my system. Running has always been a mental health lifeline, but breathing better, and being in conversation with my breath, has deepened that connection in every way.

Lottie Evans, runner and breathing coach

CHAPTER 7

Breathing assessments

How good are you at breathing? Sounds like a ridiculous question at first, but it's important to answer without guessing. We'll assess all aspects of your breathing, including mechanics, autonomic baseline, ribcage position, posture, mobility and your nasal threshold so you can be specific with where you need to focus your breath training.

'I've been breathing my whole life, mate'

'Who's the best here at breathing?' The team of athletes look a bit puzzled by the question. The deathly silence is finally broken, 'I've been doing it my whole life, Jacko!' A typically jovial response I get from at least one slightly sceptical athlete, which is not uncommon when I'm asked to start working with a group of athletes or runners. Even if it doesn't come out of your mouth, it's likely some of you reading this are at least thinking it in your heads. The scepticism is normal; I was sceptical too. I'm fit, I'm healthy and never in my 13 years of professional rugby did I feel like I had a problem with my breathing. I prided myself on being the fittest player in the team.

Rather than assuming our breathing is 'fine', we need to assess it if we want to identify the areas and weak links we can improve to turn it into what Paralympic champion and world record holder Richard Whitehead describes as his 'superpower'.

So how do we assess our breathing? I never once had my breathing assessed as a professional athlete. When I asked myself questions like, *How do I know if I'm doing it right? What does diaphragmatic breathing actually feel and look like?* I didn't have any quantifiable answers. The more I dug into it, the more I saw that breathing influenced more than just my breathing: it has knock-on effects on everything, from how your body moves to make the air come in and out (biomechanics), mobility of your spine and hips, strength of your core, the ability to stay calm and focused under pressure, and much more which we'll explore.

Alarmingly for me, when I did a number of assessments, I scored extremely poorly in every one. If that happens to be the case for you as well, do not fear. It's actually great news because they are all opportunities to get better and improve. The silver lining is that the worse you breathe at the start, the more and easier improvement you'll see. It will transform not just your running but your whole body and mind.

The following assessments look first at what I call the 'autonomic baseline': how is your breathing naturally at rest and what are your breathing habits? We finish with how your breathing behaves or misbehaves under the challenge of exercise. In the middle we look at other aspects of breathing that impact your running, such as biomechanics, ribcage posture and rib mobility, as well as further up and down the kinetic chain with spine and hip mobility.

There are a number of detailed assessments ahead. I've categorised them as:

- Basic assessments
    - Autonomic baseline
    - Biomechanical
- Going deeper
    - Ribcage and movement
    - Exercise assessment

I encourage you to use all of the assessments at the start, as they also help you to track progress as you start to train your breathing. I appreciate, though, that some of you will be, like me, itching to get started with the actual training; in which case, start with at least the basic assessments.

Basic assessments

The basic assessments cover your autonomic baseline and biomechanics of your breathing. Autonomic assessments are about your natural resting breathing habits and rhythms.

The biomechanics will be significant for those who aren't sure if they are using their diaphragm correctly, and extremely significant for runners who suffer from shallow chest breathing and things like tight hips, sore neck and tight shoulders.

Autonomic baseline assessments

There are two simple assessments I like to do with all my clients to get an understanding of what I call their autonomic baseline of breathing. They aren't directly linked to breathing during running, as they are taken at rest. But they give us a window into the auto setting, the foundation upon which we will build optimal breathing in exercise. The first is the simplest – your resting natural respiratory rate. The second is an indicator of carbon dioxide sensitivity and your psychological relationship with breathing. Both give us an indicator of nervous system regulation. For example, if someone is up-regulated, it's likely they'll have a faster respiratory rate even at rest and be more sensitive to carbon dioxide build-up and changes to their breathing cycle.

Assessment 1: Resting natural respiratory rate

This assessment is literally as simple as just counting your breaths. What's important, though, is not to change, control or alter your natural rhythm of breathing when counting it. It's actually harder than you think, because as soon as you place your attention on your breathing to start counting it, you typically start to slow it down. It's why awareness of your breathing in itself is a good practice, slowing down our breathing and helping us down-regulate when we are stressed. A 2018 study highlighted that when someone is aware of breathing and counting breathing, on average we slow it down by about 20%.[1]

For the assessment we want to know what your autonomic breathing rate and rhythm are like, so ideally you wouldn't be thinking about it, but we need you to count it to assess it.

- Have a stopwatch or set a timer for 30 seconds.
- One breath cycle is an inhale and an exhale.
- Relax, don't overthink it, and just count your breathing for 30 seconds.
- Multiply the number of breaths you took by two to give your resting respiratory rate for one minute (rather than doing it for a full minute where you're likely to slow your breathing down further).
- If you have wearable technology, like a watch that tracks heart rate, it might also give you an average of your respiratory rate so you can compare.

At rest, with a calm nervous system and efficient breathing, I like to see a respiratory rate of 10–12 breaths per minute, ideally closer to 10 if we are trying to optimise breathing for running performance.

Important things to notice during the assessment:

- Was your mouth open or closed?
- Was your tongue on the roof of the mouth naturally?
- If you were breathing with your mouth open, try redoing the assessment with your mouth closed, breathing through your nose and note if there is any difference between your respiratory rate, how you feel and tongue position.

Remember, the speed of your breathing is critical to the efficiency of your oxygen uptake from the lungs and your ability to stay relaxed when running. If you are breathing fast at rest, you're more likely to be breathing faster as soon as you start running. A breathing rate at rest of just 14, for example, doesn't seem too bad at first glance, but compared with 10 breaths/minute it's actually 40% more than you need to. That's potentially a sign of inefficiency in breathing at rest, which only gets more challenging during running. So, although to improve running performance you need to be good at breathing during running, you need a solid foundation at rest to build on.

Assessment 2: BOLT score, or control pause

The BOLT score was developed by Patrick McKeown at Oxygen Advantage from his work with the Buteyko method, where this assessment is called the control pause. It's an extremely simple assessment to perform, as you don't need any equipment or observation of yourself, apart from a watch to time how sensitive you are to carbon dioxide in your lungs.

Remember Math Roberts, the international runner out of Eryri (Snowdonia) who's won races of just one mile long and also set ultra-mountain marathon records? During our interview I was interested to try and get some objective assessment of his breathing. That wasn't going to be easy as we sat drinking coffee in a busy but cosy cafe in Llanberis. The BOLT score, however, is so simple that we were easily able to use it even in this scenario.

I explained the BOLT score, which he hadn't heard of but was more than happy to give it a go. He took a normal breath in and out, which for him naturally was through his nose at rest, slowly and gently. He pinched his nose and stopped breathing, and I started my stopwatch. We waited. We kept waiting. He had no idea what was good or not – he'd never done this assessment before. I kept waiting, I couldn't believe what I saw.

Eventually he took a breath in, but he was totally calm and appeared not to be using any willpower. The stopwatch showed 63 seconds. I blinked and took another look. Sixty-three seconds, sitting casually in the cafe after a coffee. He had no idea how good that is. When I asked him where the sensation to inhale came from, he pointed down towards his diaphragm and said, 'From my stomach.' Clearly Math Roberts is an exceptional runner over multiple distances. One thing you have to do regardless of the distance in running is a lot of breathing. Math Roberts is not only an exceptional runner, not surprisingly to me, he's also an exceptional breather.

Not that all the best runners will have the highest BOLT score, but it was similar with Richard Whitehead, who had a BOLT score of 52 seconds. BOLT is an indicator of carbon dioxide sensitivity at rest as it builds up in the lungs while you don't let it out. Obviously, it's not directly linked to running performance, but to be a strong runner, research shows that endurance athletes have a 'reduced ventilatory drive to hypercapnia',[2] meaning they are less sensitive to higher levels of carbon dioxide generated when running faster. It makes sense because they then have better control of their breathing while running. A 2024 study highlighted, however, that it's more complicated than better runners simply have a higher carbon dioxide tolerance, as this is not always the case, and a resting baseline test is very different to managing carbon dioxide while running.[3] And as we've explored, there are also other factors at play during running like mechanoreceptors and perception of effort.

So how do you do the assessment yourself? Here is how to take your BOLT score:

- Sit or lie down in a comfortable position you can relax in.
- Inhale normally then exhale normally (whatever feels natural and normal to you).
- Pause (pinch your nose, but you don't have to if it's uncomfortable) and stop breathing and start your stopwatch.
- Relax and don't overthink it.
- Wait until you get the urge to breathe in.
- Don't fight it or use any willpower. When you feel the urge to breathe in, breathe in calmly and stop the stopwatch.
- You shouldn't feel out of breath, as you weren't fighting the urge with willpower, and breathing should feel relatively normal, but not completely normal because you just paused your breathing.

The longer you can last before you feel the urge to breathe at rest, the less sensitive you are to carbon dioxide building up in the lungs and blood. Math Roberts was over one minute in a cafe after a coffee. I was less than eight seconds the first time I took it.

One of the things I've found useful as part of the observational side of this assessment is not just when you get the urge to breathe but also where in your body you feel it. Remember runner Math Roberts felt it from his diaphragm after 63 seconds. That's excellent, as we want our natural urge to be initiated from our diaphragm, as it's our primary breathing muscle. Mine initially was in my head. More like a thought; I felt a bit anxious and almost claustrophobic. That can be the case for people especially when the BOLT is low (less than 10 seconds).

It highlights an important point that breathing is not just physiological but also psychological. The fear centres in your brain are very aware of your breathing, and research has shown that being more sensitive to carbon dioxide increases your likelihood of anxiety.[4]

Initially, your BOLT score time may be lower, and the sensation to breathe comes from higher up – head (thoughts), throat, neck, chest in descending order, until the point where you have truly changed your auto and your BOLT is higher and your urge to breathe comes from lower, ideally from the diaphragm. At that point your diaphragm has come to the party on auto, and that's a very good thing!

I've worked with many professional, elite and international athletes with BOLT scores initially around 10–15 seconds, which is relatively low considering they are performing at a world-class level. They will often feel like they don't recover as well, feel more out of breath, have poor quality sleep, and when we improve their BOLT score – get them up closer to a Math Roberts – they report feeling better, less fatigued, improved recovery and sleep, as well as better breath control during performances.

Biomechanical assessments

The second section of our basics assessments is looking at breathing mechanics. With breathing mechanics, we assess how the ribcage and diaphragm are articulating in order to increase the volume of your thorax, which, remember, decreases internal pressure relative to atmospheric pressure, drawing air into the lungs.

When assessing breathing mechanics, as with the autonomic baseline assessments, we want to understand what's normal and natural. Performance physiotherapist Gemma Jefferson, who's worked with athletes taking part in multiple World, Olympic and Paralympic championships, explains, 'The most important thing with assessing breathing mechanics is the breathing assessment starts before they know you're assessing breathing. As soon as you tell someone you're assessing breathing they'll start changing it.' So, when performing these biomechanics assessments, try to breathe as normally as possible, not manipulating your normal posture or trying to breathe in a way you think is better (it may not be), to get a fair assessment of what's normal for you.

If you're a coach, try to take some visual assessments of clients' breathing habits before they realise the assessment has actually started. Sneaky, yes – but when they don't know you're assessing their breathing, that's when you get to see what their true natural habits and automation are like.

There are three types of assessments I do with clients that fall into the biomechanics category to give a well-rounded picture of how well someone can mechanically ventilate. Before we jump into the mechanics of how the ribcage and diaphragm draw air into the lungs, here's a quick reminder to use the tongue suction as an indicator of your tongue posture and airway assessment (from chapter 6). Because if the airway is compromised and airflow restricted in the airway, then your ribcage and diaphragm are affected.

Biomechanics assessment 1: Hi-Lo test – seated v supine (lying)

The Hi-Lo test is the simplest assessment of breathing mechanics to determine whether the act of ventilating is coming from a dominant upper chest expansion or a lower abdominal expansion. You'll learn in the next chapter the details of what constitutes effective and efficient biomechanics of breathing in relation to the diaphragm and ribcage synchronisation – this is just the assessment.

A 2023 study in the Journal of Strength and Conditioning Research revealed that around 91% of nearly 2000 subjects that engaged regularly in exercise were upper chest-dominant breathers, which the researchers categorise as dysfunctional.[5] So, despite this assessment being easy it's very common for people to be classified as upper chest dominant.

I suggest performing this assessment initially seated, and it can even be carried out in conjunction with when you are measuring your respiratory rate (Autonomic assessment 1).

HI-LO TEST

- Sit normally and don't adjust your posture.
- Place one hand on your upper chest and the other hand on your abdominal region.

- Use your hands to gain some external feedback on which parts of your body and ribcage are moving in order to breathe. How big is the movement and what is the direction?

Important things to notice:

- Listen to your breathing, can you hear it? Quieter breathing is slower and calmer.
- Are you breathing through your nose or mouth?
- Where is your tongue in your mouth?

If your mouth was open, close it and breathe through your nose. If you could hear your breathing, try breathing quietly. If your tongue was low down, try keeping it on the roof of your mouth and notice any difference in your breathing mechanics.

Change position: Lying down
If you felt the upper hand was moving more than the lower hand, you'll likely notice a difference when we change your body position to lying down. When you are lying down, two important things change. Your posture is likely better; as long as you are lying on a flat floor, your body is going to be flat. As you are also supported by the floor, not only are you in a better postural position to allow breathing mechanics to be easier but your diaphragm, which is a deep core stabiliser, doesn't have to stabilise you as you are fully supported, making it easier for the diaphragm to function.

Lie down on the floor and do the Hi-Lo test again. It is likely you'll notice when your diaphragm doesn't need to stabilise your trunk, as you're supported by the floor, your breathing comes from lower down and your upper chest is more relaxed.

Lying down helps you breathe better, but you don't run lying down, so one of the things you'll work on in the coming chapters is your ability to mechanically ventilate efficiently while running, rather than lying down. That will require diaphragmatic breathing and the ability to maintain stability at the same time. Get diaphragmatic breathing right while running and you'll maintain better posture, which improves running form. You'll be breathing more efficiently, which makes it easier to stay relaxed. That's smarter breathing.

Biomechanics assessment 2: Active, simulated running

Now, whether you did the Hi-Lo test seated, lying down or both, neither of those are the upright position you are in when running. Although the test gives you an insight into your breathing at rest while seated or lying, it doesn't tell us how you are likely to mechanically ventilate during exercise and running. At rest the breath is often very quiet, small and subtle, so it can be less obvious to feel what's driving it. Yet when we start running it gets challenged and exaggerated. What's driving your breathing when it's being challenged – your upper chest or your diaphragm?

The obvious thing would be to start exercising and try to feel how your ribcage and diaphragm move. But that, in practice, is actually quite difficult. When you start running, your arms swing and you can't use your hands to feel what's going on. Also, when running, each time your foot hits the floor, your body stabilises through the midline. Your intercostals, obliques and transverse abdominis all engage for stabilisation, while also being involved in breathing – so there are some confusing sensations around the abdominal region.

What's interesting is you don't actually have to run; you just need to think you're running. When assessing a client, while standing, ask them to pretend they're running at a good pace and take a few breaths as if they were running. The brain recognises that pattern and it demonstrates quite happily. Boom, we see a bigger breath and how they breathe mechanically when ventilation requirement increases. You can try this too but putting your hands on your body as in the Hi-Lo test and notice the difference.

Commonly, when simulating breathing while running, the habit of the upper chest pumping is revealed, which was perhaps hiding sneakily when assessing at rest. If you notice this happening yourself and you also get very tight shoulders and neck after running longer distances, working on your breathing mechanics will be a game changer – and that shoulder and neck pain might disappear.

Lateral expansion

The final tweak to this assessment is to switch the position of your hands from high to low and place them on the outside of the lower portion of the ribcage. This allows you to not only gauge if the breath is high or low but whether you are getting important lateral expansion of the ribcage.

Take a few more breaths where you pretend to be breathing like you're running at a good pace and, with your hands on the outside of your ribs, notice if you get any lateral expansion of the ribcage pushing the hands out.

Don'ts!
When using these active inhalations to simulate running, only perform a few breaths and then return to normal breathing. A few breaths allows you to assess your breathing when running, but if you do it a lot, you are hyperventilating rather than breathing efficiently.

It is important to notice:

- Are you breathing through your nose or mouth?
- How noisy is your breathing? The more you can hear your breathing, the faster and less in control of it you'll be; and the faster and noisier it is, the more prone you are to inefficient shallow upper chest breathing.
- If you close your mouth and slow your breathing down, making it a little quieter but still taking big breaths as if running so you can feel the movement, do you notice any difference in how your ribcage expands?

Biomechanics assessment 3: Diaphragm activation test (DAT)

This is one of my favourite assessments because I see it as one of the most important. Also, it not only acts as an assessment of your ability to activate your diaphragm but also helps as a simple exercise to activate it better.

In the next chapter we look at how the brain has to send a signal via the phrenic nerve to your diaphragm for it to contract. This can be totally automatic in good diaphragmatic breathers, or it can feel completely alien or almost impossible to those who have upper chest-dominated compensatory breathing patterns.

I first came across this during a training course with Dr Cobb from Z Health Performance, who described it as a 'blocked inhalation'. It was an absolute game changer for me because I was finally able to answer the question of what my diaphragm feels like when it contracts. I'm excited for you to feel it too!

> **DAT ASSESSMENT**
> - Take a normal breath in and out of the nose, then pinch your nose.
> - Hold your breath – don't let any air in.
> - Try to initiate a strong inhale while you're 'blocking your airway'; in other words, holding your breath and not letting any air in.

If you can activate your diaphragm when you try to breathe in, you'll feel a pulse or contraction of your diaphragm as though it wants to jump out of your stomach. That's because when you try to breathe in, the diaphragm ideally should contract and in doing so move down and flatten out. But because you're holding your breath it can't move as there is no air coming in, so it contracts isometrically instead. Isometric contractions are great for helping to activate muscles, which is why this is not just an important assessment. It is also a simple exercise you can use to improve your ability to activate your diaphragm and improve the neural firing down your phrenic nerve to the diaphragm from your brain. You need to be able to consciously contract your diaphragm before it's going to happen unconsciously when running.

If you felt nothing or just your chest, shoulders or neck trying to lift up, don't worry, you're not on your own. But it is very important to change that activation pattern for your inhalation with the exercises demonstrated in the next chapter.

Dos and don'ts!
It is important to remember that tongue position influences the function of the diaphragm, so have your tongue at the roof of the mouth when activating the diaphragm, as we learned from Dr Lomas.

Going deeper
For those of us keen to take a deeper dive into understanding breathing – and how it affects not just your performance but your movement and

mobility – or for those seeking to reduce hip pain and wondering if breathing plays a part, these next assessments go deeper.

Ribcage and movement assessments

These assessments look at the ribcage itself, the positioning of it, the effect on your posture and mobility of the ribcage itself, as well as the spine and hips. A really important aspect of breathing, which is often surprising but essential for runners, is how your ribcage position and posture affects your breathing and vice versa.

The position of your ribcage directly affects diaphragm function[6] and, consequently, your running posture, which is why I view it as an important part of the breathing assessments. All of your ribs connect into the vertebrate of your thoracic spine, so how you breathe and how your ribs move affect your thoracic spine, which, again, is important for good running posture. As the thoracic spine is a junction for the vagus nerve, when we open up the posterior (back) portion of the ribcage, not only do we create freedom in our spine and breathing, we also open up other areas of the body. What is particularly helpful for runners is the effect it has on the hips. You'll learn the breathing mobilisations in chapter 9, which will transform the mobility of your spine and hips, potentially alleviating hip pain. I've seen it be a real game changer for many runners of all levels.

The initial part of this assessment is finding the starting point of your ribcage in relation to the movement of your spine and pelvis.

RIBCAGE ASSESSMENT

- Lie flat on the floor with legs straight and body relaxed.
- While relaxed and supported by the floor, determine the resting position of your ribcage in relation to your spine and pelvis.
- Use your hands to feel the front of your body. How much can you feel your lower ribs? Are they sticking up out of your t-shirt or do they feel relatively flat?
- Place your hand underneath your lower back and feel how arched it is.

If your ribs at the front felt like they were sticking up out of your t-shirt like a triceratops, you'll likely notice that the back feels overly arched too. That's because the ribs wrap around your body. The ribs at the front are the same ribs you feel at the back. If the front is sticking up, so are the ones at the back, making your back arched more. This will impact the extent you can use your diaphragm, because the diaphragm is attached to those lower ribs. The effect it has on your pelvis affects the tightness in your hip flexors and hamstrings, as well as the ability to get into a good tall posture for improved running form.

Often the tightness and stiffness we generate in the kinetic chain from lots of running means the ribcage is often pushed forward and tilted back, and you'll notice ribs sticking up and your back overly arched when lying flat. If that's the case, don't worry, we have the 'fix' for that with breathing mobilisation covered in chapter 9.

INFRA-STERNAL ANGLE

Checking your infra-sternal angle — the angle your two lowest ribs make with your sternum (breastbone) — is also part of our ribcage assessment. It's easiest to do this in front of a mirror so you can see what is happening or video it to watch back. You are looking at whether the angle the ribs make with the sternum is even from left to right, and whether it is narrow, wide or neutral. Neutral would be around 45 degrees, so the total would be 90 degrees.

- As you inhale, the angle should open up and get wider as the ribs laterally expand moving up and out.
- As you exhale, they should move back down and in, and the angle reduces.
- If the resting angle is less than 90 degrees in total, it's deemed to be narrow.
- If it's greater than 90 degrees, it is wider than normal.

Dos and don'ts

It's important to say our skeletons are all slightly different; we aren't looking for perfect symmetry or the 'perfect' 90-degree angle (like we see

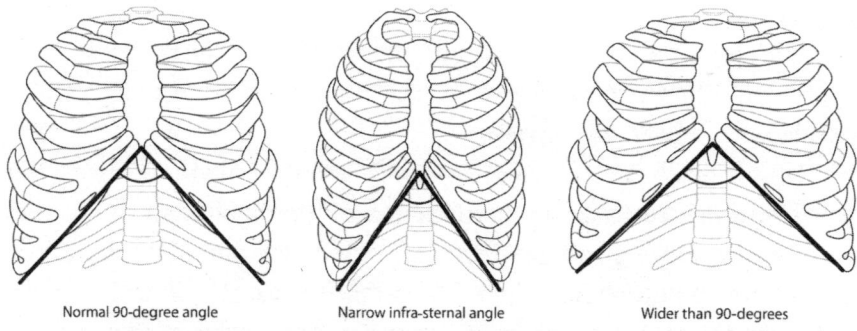

Normal 90-degree angle   Narrow infra-sternal angle   Wider than 90-degrees

The angle and position of your ribs can effect the function of your diaphragm

in textbooks). Everyone has their normal differences and there are some specific differences between males and females that I'll cover in the next section. As we come in all different shapes and sizes, so do our ribcages, so don't freak out if yours isn't 'perfect' or symmetrical – it doesn't necessarily mean it's wrong or needs altering. However, being aware allows you to try some of the breathing mobilisations from chapter 9 in a way that's specific to your ribcage to see if it makes any improvements to how you feel, breathe and run.

A common phrase thrown around about the ribcage is 'rib flare', associated with being stuck in an 'open' or extension pattern. This would be the ribs lifted up and out. If you were lying on your back, you could feel or see the lowest ribs sticking up out of the t-shirt. An assumption is that if we see the back arched, with the ribcage forward in an extension position, then the ribs would be flared (wide infra-sternal angle), which we can see, but this is not always the case. Because not only do we have the ribs themselves in relation to the sternum, we also have to consider the position of the entire ribcage.

The ribcage can be in what I'd describe as projected forward and also tilted back (posteriorly tilted), meaning the back would be arched, the ribs would be sticking up and in an extension position, but the infra-sternal angle can still be narrow. So just because someone is arched in the back with the ribs up, don't assume it's a rib flare and that the infra-sternal angle will be wide, as it may not be.

With runners, especially those who run shorter distances and more powerfully due to posterior chain development for speed work, it's common to see an arched back and anterior pelvic tilt that results in a 'projected forward' ribcage. However, the infra-sternal angle can be unrelated to this, in my experience.

If the ribcage is projected forward, it's out of alignment with the pelvis and this restricts the full function of the diaphragm. If the ribs are sticking out in a 'rib flare', this too will restrict the function of the diaphragm and the ability of the ribs themselves to articulate effectively. If the ribs are sticking out they keep the diaphragm stretched and don't allow it to relax on the exhale. Rib flare also means that an exhalation will be harder (as they have to move back in), and even the inhale itself can be restricted as the ribs can't start moving out effectively on the inhale if they are already stuck out. It's often described as 'being stuck in an inhalation position'; it's hard to inhale if your ribs are already expanded and it restricts the ribs moving in on an exhale.

Movement assessments: Ribcage, spine and hips

If your ribs don't move, your spine won't move, as they join at the thoracic spine. So assessing your ability to rotate through your thoracic spine is a great indicator of your thoracic mobility and also your rib mobility and freedom in your ribcage as a whole.

THORACIC ROTATION

- Kneel on the floor with your bottom as close to your heels as comfortably possible.
- Place one elbow on the floor in front of the knee on the same side, in contact with the knee, with your palm flat on the floor to steady you. This position helps to 'fix your hips' so that you only rotate from your thoracic spine and ribcage.
- Place the other hand on the back of the head.
- Try to rotate up and around as far as you can comfortably.
- Notice where you feel tight and restricted in the movement, and if you film yourself doing it, you'll be able to see the range you achieve.

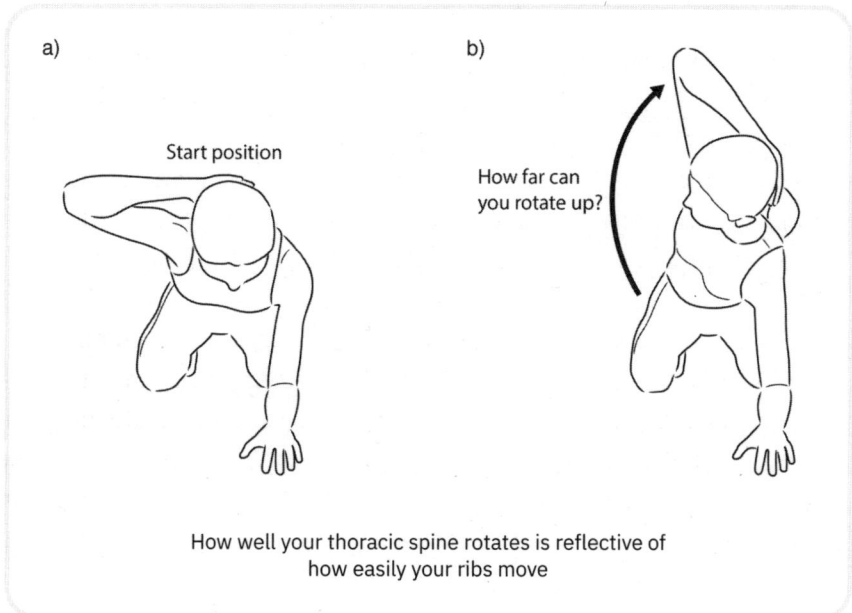

How well your thoracic spine rotates is reflective of how easily your ribs move

Hip mobility

As your diaphragm connects through the fascia to the muscles related to your hips, particularly psoas major and quadratus lumborum, how you breathe can have a direct impact on your hip range of motion. That's because tightness in your diaphragm will affect tightness in muscles like psoas major (hip flexor) which can pull the pelvis into an anterior pelvic tilt (rolled forward). When the pelvis position is compromised it can affect all movement at the hip joint, not just hip flexion. For example, the hamstrings can feel tighter as they are attached at the back of the pelvis, and when the pelvis is rolled forward the hamstrings are lengthened and increased in tension.

How often do runners complain of tight hip flexors, adductors (groin) and tight hamstrings and we blame it on running and not doing our stretches? You'll learn in chapter 9 from performance physiotherapist Gemma Jefferson that it might be your breathing that's the root cause of your tight hips. I'll also show you the breathing mobilisation to help free them!

For now, we are just assessing the range of motion in your hips. There are many ways you can assess flexion, extension, abduction, adduction, and external and internal rotation at the hip, but I like to keep things as simple as possible. So, we're going to do two very straightforward things.

ASSESS HIPS AND HAMSTRINGS

The first is to simply stand up with relatively straight legs, just a soft bend at the knee if that's more comfortable (just make sure you keep it the same when you do a retest), and reach down towards your toes to see how close you are to touching them. Most of us are so tight in our glutes and our hamstrings as runners that we are way off touching our toes. A social runner in his sixties said, 'Jacko, I've never been able to touch my toes, mate,' but after a few of the breathing mobilisations from chapter 9 and no stretching at all, he touched his toes while standing for the first time in just a matter of minutes. Breathing works, and your diaphragm affects your hip flexors and your hip flexors affect your hamstrings.

Assess hip internal and external rotation

The other assessment for your hips is how well it rotates in the socket, both internally and externally. Both internal and external hip rotation are often tight with runners; they're important for good movement and healthy hips. Loosen off these bad boys with some of the breathing mobilisation exercises, and not only might your hip or back pain that you've been putting up with for years finally subside, but the freedom in your hips and pelvis can help improve your stride length and running form.

ASSESS HIP INTERNAL AND EXTERNAL ROTATION

- Lie on the floor on your back, long and relaxed with one leg completely straight.
- Bend the other leg at 90 degrees and flex your hip, bringing your knee towards you so that the thigh bone (femur) is vertical.
- Hold the thigh in that vertical position with your hands.

- With the knee bent at 90 degrees, try to rotate your foot to the outside. If it's your right foot, try to rotate it out to the right. See how far it gets, where it feels tight and how it feels. This is your internal hip rotation. Yes, the foot is going to the outside, but your femur is internally rotated in your hip socket.
- In the same position, rotate the foot the other way. The foot comes inwards towards your centre line. If this is your right foot, it's moving towards the left across your body. This is external hip rotation.
- Swap and do the same on the other leg.

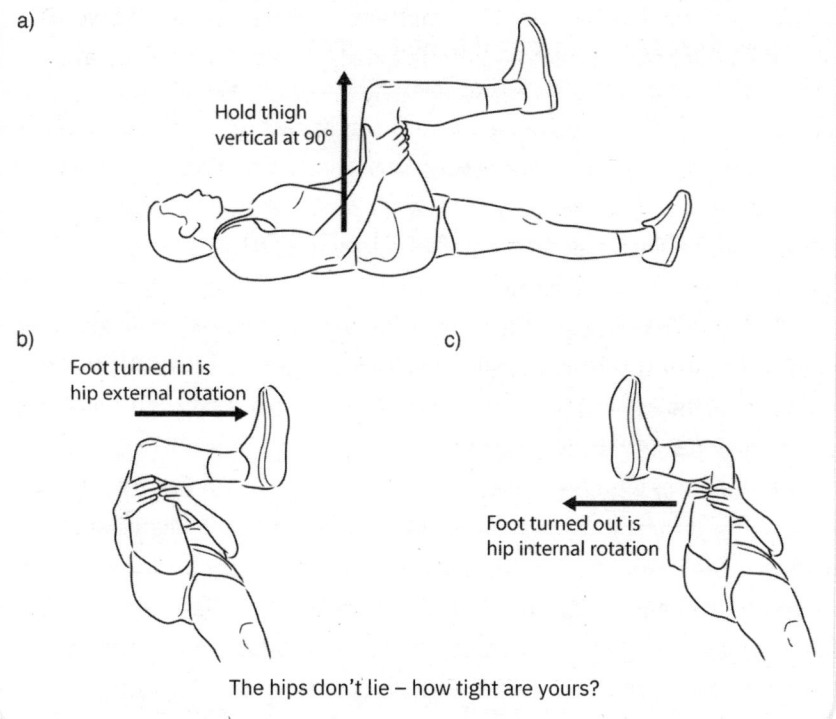

The hips don't lie – how tight are yours?

You could measure the angles if you really wanted to get quantitative with data, but it's not necessary. Most people see and feel a big difference once they've worked through the breathing mobilisations in the next chapter. Personally, I like to take a before and after picture or video to be able to see the difference – putting it on Instagram is optional! But tag me if you do: @thebreathrunningcoach.

Important to note: being aware of what is normal for you is important for these assessments so you can detect when you're getting tight and stiff in a particular area and address it before it becomes a problem or leads to injury. It's normal to notice that one leg or one side is tighter than the other, that's fine, but you might benefit from balancing them out by focusing on specific mobilisations in the next chapter. Getting familiar by using them as simple test and retest assessments gives you a better idea about how your body is actually feeling and moving on a regular basis – as well as a nice way to check progress.

Exercise assessment: Nasal threshold (NT)

The final assessment is different from all previous assessments because it's performed during exercise rather than at rest. It's a really important one because its focus is about how you are able to breathe, manage airflow, carbon dioxide and recovery during exercise. All parameters that will improve when you integrate the advice from this book into your training. This is you getting a baseline.

This assessment uses the nose to provide resistance to test out your diaphragm and other respiratory muscles along with carbon dioxide levels in the blood and lungs compared with normal mouth breathing. It assesses your current NT during exercise.

The point at which you switch from nose to mouth breathing during increasing running intensity can be closely linked to ventilatory and lactate thresholds, as seen from my own VO_2 max testing. We don't have to do all of our running breathing nasally, but this assessment lets us know what our current capacity is. It's something that will improve and increase with time, and the nose can be a great training tool for strengthening your diaphragm, carbon dioxide tolerance, regulating your breathing and heart rate, and improving your recovery.

Professor George Dallam explained to me that you can test your own relatively easily: 'Perform similar to a graded exercise test, gradually increase the intensity over a certain time interval and keep doing that until you can't go any faster (with your nose)... the point you are feeling extreme air hunger you are probably truly hypoventilation (under-breathing), which is just your sensation as a subjective marker, but it gives you an idea.'

To perform this assessment, you could run indoors on a treadmill, which is often easiest for controlling things like pace, but it could be done outside, just try to have a relatively flat area to run on. It could even be done on an indoor bike or assault bike in a gym (but obviously running is more specific for runners).

NASAL THRESHOLD (NT)

- After a five-minute gentle warm-up, you are going to measure your heart rate (if possible) and running pace (if on an exercise bike, RPM or watts), gradually increasing the intensity in 30-second increments.
- Start with a very easy pace for the first 30 seconds.
- Every 30 seconds increase the pace slightly and maintain that pace for the 30-second period.
- Keep doing this until you reach the point where you cannot maintain nasal breathing any longer and have to switch to mouth breathing – aiming to reach your maximum capacity in around five minutes or so.
- At that switch point make a note of what your pace and heart rate are (if you wanted to know what per cent of your maximum it was, you could continue with mouth breathing until you literally can't run or cycle any faster).
- Time 90 seconds of recovery to see how much your heart rate comes down from its peak at the end of the test when you switched to mouth breathing. Make a note of your peak heart rate and after those 90 seconds of recovery.

After implementing the breath-training strategies in the rest of this book, when you retest your NT and your heart rate recovery, you'll be surprised. You'll see how much more you can do with your nose, how good it can feel (I know it often doesn't at the start), how much faster you can recover your heart rate and how you feel when you know how to use your breathing optimally.

Differences for females

It's important to be aware of some biological differences between men and women that affect breathing. Speaking with Catherine Jackson, physiologist and health coach, working with female professional and international athletes across a number of sports, she passionately outlines some considerations: 'Let's acknowledge the existence of physiological differences between males and females, in order to better understand ourselves, as active females.' She explains that women's bodies are not simply a smaller version of male bodies. 'Research shows the female hearts and lungs are smaller versus males, even when adjusting for size and weight.[7] Their structure and function also differ, with lung shape and rib orientation, as well as narrower airways being different.[8] A female red blood cell count is lower, with lower haemoglobin levels (which carries the oxygen to the working muscles).[9] All of which reduces oxygen-carrying capacity.'

When we look at how this translates in practice, research suggests that during submaximal intensities, women report increased breathlessness and perceived exertion at equivalent intensities compared with men of similar fitness levels. Evidence indicates a 'higher neural respiratory drive',[10] meaning the signals sent from the brain to the respiratory muscles to initiate breathing are stronger, experienced as a greater effort to breathe.[11]

Whenever the drive to breathe is increased, women have to go bigger and/or faster compared with men. In previous studies, women were more likely to adopt a more shallow and rapid breathing pattern, which, as we've seen, is less efficient.[12] Catherine explained: 'Females appear to be more susceptible to respiratory system limitations during exercise versus men. So I believe we stand to benefit more so, from specifically training our breathing.' Other big differences between males and females are the hormones involved in the female reproductive cycle, namely oestrogen and progesterone, which affects all systems, not just the reproductive system. Catherine explained the role of those hormones and noted that they affect 'the heart, brain, our emotions, immune system, energy production, temperature regulation, bones, muscles and much more! A female's life stage will mean changes in these areas too.'

Progesterone (which affects carbon dioxide sensitivity) causes an increase in breathing.[13] If ovulation occurs, progesterone reaches a peak in the mid-luteal phase (around a week before the start of a period), which can contribute to breathlessness. It can also have an effect on heart rate variability (HRV), a measure of autonomic nervous system (ANS) function.[14] The resulting impact being that female athletes notice cyclical differences in perception of pain, level of exertion and capacity to recover.

Finally, Catherine explains: 'Currently there's probably not enough strong evidence to allow these findings to dictate your training but certainly tuning into your menstrual cycle, especially if/when you ovulate and understanding how you feel in exercise during the different phases of your cycle is recommended. Clients anecdotally feel better doing more challenging sessions during the first half of the cycle, usually after their main bleeding days, and focus more on easier sessions and more recovery around the progesterone peak into the bleeding days.'

Catherine highlights some key differences that are important to understand and appreciate when assessing breathing as a female, and how they may impact breathing sensations and exercise performance not just during an assessment but also in exercise as a whole.

We can hopefully now answer the question: *How do I know if I'm breathing right?* Breathing is multidimensional and we have objective assessments, which provide an insight into your current baseline, a window into how good your breathing is or how much opportunity you have to improve. It will also give you some clues as to what areas to focus on. We'll also use them regularly to retest, allowing us to track our progress – it's always a nice boost, or as we used to say at rugby 'a bum tap', to see how much you've improved.

It's time to do an assessment of your baseline, and then we can get to work!

Key takeaways

- Your breathing at rest provides an indication of both your breathing efficiency and regulation of nervous system (how stressed you are).
- Getting a baseline of your assessment at the start is helpful for identifying areas to improve and track progress, which is good for motivation.
- How you breathe affects how you move and your posture, especially the spine and hips.
- If your ribs don't move, your spine can't move, which limits not just your breathing but your running posture.

I have been following Jacko's programme for a while, and I have benefited in many ways. I suffer with chronic silent reflux, and I was very conscious how my symptoms were triggered during exercise. I would hyperventilate during my workouts, and this would affect my performance.

Following Jacko's programming I have learned how to manage my breathing during exercise and how to use the training to recover faster. My running, my exercise performance and my overall well-being have improved since I started training my breathing. I am seeing so many benefits and I am very excited to see where this journey takes me.

Michaela Pugh, Crossfit athlete

CHAPTER 8

Unlock the power of your diaphragm

I believe breathing is a skill. Elite fell runner Ellis Bland told us earlier that most runners have a gross misunderstanding of what good breathing is. Like any skill, you can get better at it. You just need to know how to do it. With breathing, the key relationship is between your ribcage and diaphragm.

Let me introduce you to your new best friend . . .

'Does the diaphragm contract on an inhale or an exhale?' I asked the group during a workshop back in 2023, and they all looked a bit puzzled, even slightly intimidated. I hope it wasn't the way I asked the simple question. Eventually a few of them realised it was a 50–50 answer. I encouraged them to just have a guess, and one slightly more confident coach, with his hands on his stomach region, exhaled strongly, felt his abdomen tense and shouted out 'exhale'. A few others saw what he did and nodded along, saying 'yeah, the exhale'. A quieter lady in the corner looked a bit puzzled and said, 'I thought the diaphragm contracts on an inhale?' I tried to bring some order to the chaos and asked for a show of hands. 'Who thinks it contracts on an inhale?' Just a few hands went up, 'And who thinks it contracts on an exhale?' The majority of the hands went up. The majority were wrong.

Where is the diaphragm? What does diaphragmatic breathing look and feel like? They were the next two questions I asked the group. 'Is it belly breathing?' someone answered slightly tentatively, as everyone felt like the diaphragm contraction question should have been an easy one. Belly breathing is going in the right direction, with lower breathing mechanics rather than upper chest-dominant breathing. The diaphragm, however, is not in your belly and the lungs are not in your belly, and that is obviously where the air needs to go when we inhale.

It seems like we could all benefit from some breathing education, starting with diaphragm and its many roles.

The many roles of the diaphragm

The diaphragm has been identified as possibly 'the most important muscle in the human body'.[1] It's not just a breathing muscle, although that's a key part of its role. When we get it right, 'diaphragmatic breathing is correlated with various positive health benefits, including reduced resting heart rate, post-exercise oxidative stress, increased postural control, and baroreflex sensitivity'.[2]

The word diaphragm is actually derived from the Greek word *diáphragma,* meaning partition. According to James Earls, author of *Born to Walk,* the diaphragm's first role during human evolution was to act as a barrier between your lungs and your organs to protect them and stop them moving around too much inside of you. With the central position of the diaphragm as that 'partition', it can be a key player in postural stabilisation, which is very important for runners. It is, in fact, the largest of our deep core muscles. When it's not working correctly, there's a knock-on effect to the other muscles around our trunk and hips, which have to compensate for the lack of stability if the diaphragm isn't creating it through our breathing dynamics. Other musculature tightens up around the hips and won't 'turn off', creating excessive tension in our hip flexors, for example. So much so that performance physiotherapist Gemma Jefferson, who we heard from in the last chapter, explained that if an athlete is struggling with hip pain and she has identified that they're upper chest-dominant breathers, until she resolves the diaphragmatic breathing pattern, the hip issue won't go away. Are your hips tight from running? Have you ever worked on your diaphragm? You might get significant relief in those hips when we get your diaphragm happier.

It doesn't stop there; the diaphragm is also a lymphatic pump. The pressure changes it creates within the body – which not only allows air to move into the lungs on an inhale as the diaphragm contracts and moves down – also helps with lymph flow. Dr Perry Nickleston, a pioneer in the world of lymphatics, explains, 'the diaphragm plays a crucial role in detoxification.' Similar to its function as a lymphatic pump, the diaphragm massages your internal organs, helping to provide good blood flow to those organs and improving vital processes such as digestion.

The vagus nerve, the 10th cranial nerve, often described as the 'wandering nerve' because it branches out from the brain stem and visits all of the major organs, is also influenced by the diaphragm. On its journey around the body, it passes directly through the diaphragm and plays a vital role in feeding information back to the brain about the state of our internal environment. The vagus nerve is instrumental with the ANS, governs HRV and good vagal tone (essentially, when the vagus nerve is 'happy' and functioning well, it sends good quality information back to the brain about the internal physiological state of the body) is critical for parasympathetic processes that occur during recovery, which we cover in detail in chapter 12.

Because the vagus nerve passes directly through the diaphragm, they have an important relationship we can influence through correct diaphragmatic breathing. This relationship can affect not just how efficiently we breathe but our ability to relax and even the way we transfer force as our foot hits the ground through the stability the diaphragm can help create.

Hence why athletes feed back: 'It's a total game changer, Jacko,' when they finally start to get to grips with this key player.

There are two major aspects to optimising diaphragmatic breathing. The first is the diaphragm itself and how it moves and functions. The second is the positioning of the diaphragm, as it's 'housed' within the bottom of the ribcage.

Anatomy and function

Firstly, let's clarify that the diaphragm contracts on an inhale and relaxes on an exhale. During inspiration, a message to breathe in (neurons) is sent from the respiratory centres in the brain stem via the phrenic nerve to the inspiratory muscles, mainly the diaphragm and external intercostal muscles.

To be fair to me and anyone else who finds the diaphragm a somewhat strange muscle, its anatomy is a little confusing for a couple of reasons. It's deep inside so we can't easily feel it, flex it or see it, like your bicep. It's also a very strange shape compared with more linear muscles, such as the biceps, which when they shorten, simply flex your elbow.

Author of *Body by Breath* Jill Miller has been studying anatomy and movement for over 30 years and is an expert when it comes to breathing, especially the diaphragm. During an interview on my podcast 'Between Breaths' she explained, 'The diaphragm's origin and insertion actually swap halfway through its contraction,' which is unlike any other muscle. This was mind-blowing to hear, but it explains why there is confusion around the contraction of the diaphragm and what it feels like. She went on to explain the diaphragm has very few sensory neurons compared with other muscles, which is why the movement of it feels much more alien compared with your bicep, for example, which has more sensory neurons and contracts in only one linear direction.

The shape of the diaphragm can be likened to a parachute. However, as we are seeing with this complex muscle, it's not that simple. The diaphragm is double domed, so there is a left hemisphere (slightly smaller) and a right hemisphere (slightly bigger), which makes matters worse, as it's not even symmetrical. It feels like the diaphragm wants to confuse us. But when we understand how it's designed and meant to function in optimal breathing, things start to make a whole lot more sense. It also feels really great to breathe how we're designed to, from a functional anatomy perspective. Ultimately, breathing efficiently not only feels better, it requires less effort and uses less energy and oxygen to actually breathe when running, meaning you can relax, as energy and oxygen can go to your legs instead.

Meet your diaphragm and its home, your ribcage

Let's now locate one of the most important muscles in your body. Your diaphragm attaches both centrally to the spine and peripherally to the ribcage. It's very important to appreciate the diaphragm is not in your belly (we'll get to belly breathing later). So many people I meet, just like me at the start, don't realise where their ribcage and diaphragm are in relation to their body.

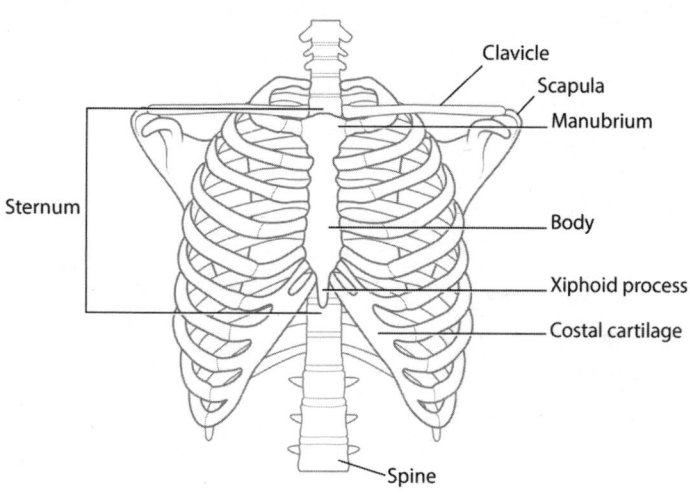

The 'home' where your diaphragm and lungs live

TRY THIS

Understand how big your ribcage is and where your diaphragm is within it.

- Find your left collar bone with your right hand and place a finger on it.
- With your left hand locate your sternum (breastbone) and follow your lowest left rib diagonally down towards your hip.
- Notice how low your lowest rib goes.
- Keep your hand on your lowest rib and appreciate how big your ribcage is, when you know your first rib (highest rib) is just above your collar bone.

Your ribcage is massive, your entire trunk is basically your ribcage and your trunk is almost all of you! You just have your arms hanging off the sides and your pelvis and legs hanging off the bottom! Our diaphragm is housed in the bottom of your ribcage. So, feel it by tracking your fingers along the two lowest ribs on each side of the sternum. Your diaphragm attaches to these lowest ribs, as well as the lumbar spine.

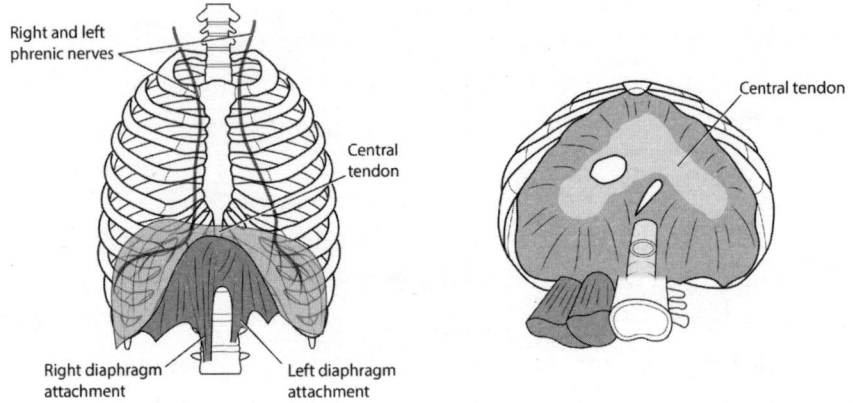

One of the most important muscles in your body: your diaphragm

During efficient diaphragmatic breathing, when we inhale, the role of the diaphragm is to descend downwards (inferiorly) into the abdominal cavity, which increases the vertical diameter of the thorax, thereby increasing volume. Similarly, there should be an increase in volume created by the lateral movement of the ribs to facilitate the movement of the diaphragm, via contraction of the external intercostal muscles. As the diaphragm moves downwards from the central tendon contracting, it occupies the space within itself due to the domed shape – the central part moving down and the sides moving out. The diaphragm attaches to the cartilages of ribs 7 to 10 and directly to floating ribs 11 and 12; as the diaphragm descends downwards during its contraction, the widening of these ribs by the external intercostal muscles facilitates this space for the diaphragm to move. The external intercostal muscles connect adjacent to the ribs and run in an orientation sloping down and forwards, so as they contract, the ribs are pulled up and out, like bucket handles on either side of you, expanding the ribcage.

The key is that the ribs are moving up and out (like bucket handles on either side) in synchronisation as the diaphragm is moving down like a pump. The distance the diaphragm moves downwards is known as the 'zone of apposition' (ZOA), which, at rest, can be as little as just 1cm when breathing is calm and efficient. During intense exercise the total excursion of the diaphragm can reach up to 10cm.[3] But if your ribcage and intercostal muscles are tight and your diaphragm is all jacked up (tight and restricted), you're fighting a losing battle during running to increase your ZOA to increase tidal volume like the elites.

When the diaphragm contracting and the lower ribcage expanding initiate this movement, it means air is 'pulled' into the lower portions of the lungs. This is beneficial as it's where the great density of alveoli are in the lungs, and where there's the most blood due to gravity. In his book *West's Respiratory Physiology*, expert John West emphasises that not all regions of the lung are equal: 'The lower regions of the lung ventilate better than the upper zones'.[4] If the expansion of the ribcage is driven by the upper chest accessory breathing muscles (scalenes, sternocleidomastoid) as a compensatory pattern, then the air is drawn into the upper portion of the lungs more than the lower lobes. This can happen at a faster rate because there is less distance for the air to travel, which, as we've learned, is less efficient. We want the air to get into the lower regions of the lungs, and the movement of the lower ribs and diaphragm are essential to this.

It's not just about inhales

Is an inhale more important than an exhale? Inhales typically get more of our attention, but is that fair? The quality and size of your inhale affects the quality and size of your exhale, and vice versa. Breathing is circular, and each part influences the other. Most people make the same mistake that I did at the start: we focus purely on the inhale and we're missing 50% of the breathing cycle. That 50% (the exhale) that we overlook affects both the positioning of the ribcage and the starting point of the next inhale.

A 2022 study noted that we have specific mechanoreceptors in the chest wall, diaphragm and intercostals that help our understanding of where our ribcage is positioned and how it's expanding, but too often we are simply unaware.[5] Other studies have shown that training our awareness helps to improve breathing mechanics, so, importantly, with practice we can improve.[6]

At rest, exhalation is passive, relying on the natural elasticity in the lungs, ribcage ligament tissue and the fascia of the diaphragm. During exercise, exhalation becomes gradually more active to meet the metabolic demands of the exercise, with the active exhalation initiated by muscles of the abdomen wall contracting, mainly the rectus abdominis, internal and external obliques, and transverse abdominis. During contraction of these muscles of the abdominal wall, intra-abdominal pressure increases, pushing the diaphragm upwards.[7] The internal intercostal muscles help to bring the ribs downwards and inwards on active exhalations, and carbon dioxide is offloaded from the blood via the lungs as we exhale.

When we exhale, the movement downwards and inwards (flexion and internal rotation) of the ribs is essential to allow the diaphragm to move back up. If the ribcage and the ribs themselves are tight and 'stuck', the diaphragm is compromised. This can occur when the muscles between the ribs (external and internal intercostal muscles) are tight, as well as other surrounding muscles that attach directly to the ribs, like pectoralis minor and serratus anterior. The ribs themselves also have joints as they articulate with the vertebrae in the thoracic spine. The joints can also become tight and restrict the movement of the ribs.

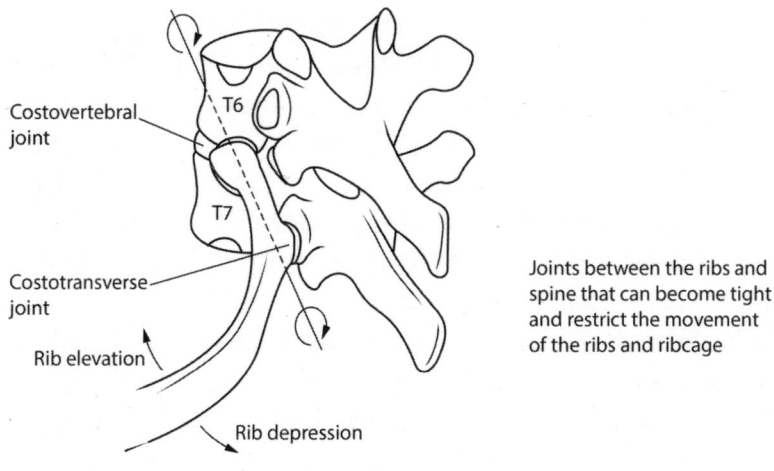

When the ribs don't move, the spine won't move – because they are jointed at the thoracic spine

So many athletes I work with – whether an international athlete or an amateur parkrunner – have tight ribs and weak exhalations to begin with because they can't get their ribs down and in. It doesn't just restrict the exhale; it affects the next inhale and the position of the entire ribcage. If you can't exhale well, you'll find more intense running even harder due to the increased amount of carbon dioxide that the body is generating, as you can't get rid of it efficiently with weak exhalations. Working on the mobility of the lower ribs, as well as the activation and strength of these exhalation muscles, is hugely beneficial for runners, and I've got the perfect exercise for you (see page 156 – exhale floor bridge exercise).

Position of the ribcage

The position of the ribcage is critical to the function of the diaphragm. This was highlighted in a 2019 study that compared two breathing postures – hands on knees versus hands on head – to compare the effects on diaphragm function and recovery heart rates.[8] The study noted that hands on knees improved the function of the diaphragm by increasing the ZOA and therefore tidal volume and volume of carbon dioxide that athletes could exhale. This led to improved heart rate recovery times during high-intensity interval training.

The study shows two key things – firstly the effort of the ribcage position on the diaphragm, and secondly the strength of the diaphragm itself. Both of which impact our ability to optimise ventilation. When the ribcage position is compromised, the diaphragm becomes restricted and we see a reduction in ZOA and resultant tidal volume. The more compromised position was hands on head, as tightness in the thoracic spine and shoulders saw a compensation of arching the back and rolling the pelvis forward (anterior pelvic tilt). This position projects the ribcage forward, bringing the diaphragm with it, creating misalignment with the pelvis. In contrast, having the spine more neutral with ribcage stacked on top of the pelvis (the hands-on-knees posture) improved the function of the diaphragm and volume of air they could breathe. The final point to note is when you are bent over with hands on knees, you are supporting yourself. Your diaphragm doesn't have to work so hard for postural stabilisation, so it can focus more on its role as a breathing muscle, which means inhaling large volumes is easier. If you were lying down it would be easier still, hence why the practical exercises at the end of this chapter start in a lying position when we are learning.

But when you are running, you aren't supported, so not only do we need good ribcage position, we also need a strong diaphragm to both stabilise us and draw sufficient air into the lungs. Like all muscles, the diaphragm functions better when it's stronger. So, don't skip diaphragm day, bro!

> **TRY THIS**
>
> **Feel the effect of your ribcage on your diaphragm yourself**
> - Lie flat on the floor with your legs straight.
> - Arch your back, roll your pelvis forwards and push your ribcage towards the ceiling as much as you can to compromise your diaphragm.
> - Take the biggest breath in you can and feel the restriction of your diaphragm.
> - Compare that with lying flat with knees bent and feet flat (semi-supine) with spine in neutral and ribcage aligned with the pelvis.
> - Take the biggest breath in you can and feel the difference!

Finally, as we're about to jump into the exercises to learn and practise correct diaphragmatic breathing, here's a reminder not to assume you're doing it well just because it's automatic – as well as some encouragement of the gains you can expect to see. We know by now that a diaphragmatic breath takes longer because the air has further to travel, but a 2022 study found that 'increasing tidal volume with slower breathing doesn't necessarily cue diaphragmatic breathing'.[9]

Diaphragmatically breathing might not just happen on its own because you're slowing your breathing down and trying to control it. I said at the start that I see breathing as a skill – we need some practice. One study saw endurance runners improve breathing efficiency over a two-month period by increasing tidal volume and reducing breathing rate by practising diaphragmatic breathing for at least 10 minutes five times per week. They reduced breathing rates on average from 59 breaths per minute to 52, an 11% reduction, and tidal volume increased by over 10%.[10] Slower breathing but larger breaths. Essentially, breathing more like an elite runner by using the power of their diaphragm.

Let's start doing the same for you!

Diaphragm and biomechanics exercises

To start harnessing the power of our diaphragm to breathe more like the elites, I will guide you through my three favourite breathing mechanics exercises. These involve firstly being able to activate your diaphragm, and then progress to engaging the correct movements of the ribs on both the inhale and the often-overlooked important exhale.

By the end of these three exercises, we'll have the foundations in place for correct diaphragmatic breathing, which include:

- Alignment and stacking ribcage
- Role of the diaphragm
- Articulation of ribs

Starting position – why supine?

We've learned the role of the diaphragm is both for ventilation and postural stability. Therefore, when trying to address the ventilatory aspect of its function, we want to position and support the body to reduce the diaphragm's 'job' of postural stability – basically make its life easier!

The semi-supine position (lying on your back, knees bent and feet flat) allows for the spine and mid-section to be supported to offload the diaphragm's role to stabilise you. With knees bent and feet flat, it also helps to position your ribcage and pelvis in good alignment. It's not the end point, as we'll see – we need to be able to breathe well biomechanically while running. But it's a good place to start and learn.

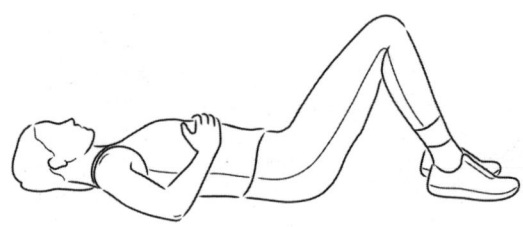

Align your ribcage and pelvis, while making the diaphragm's job easier in the semi-supine position

Exercise: Blocked inhale

I struggled to answer what it feels like to contract the diaphragm until the first time I performed a blocked inhalation and it lit up! Remember the blocked inhalation from the diaphragm activation test (DAT) in the last chapter? We can use it as an exercise to help activate the diaphragm. It's the first piece of the puzzle and the most important because if you can't activate it, you can't improve its function.

One of the most effective ways to help feel a muscle contraction is to perform an isometric muscle contraction. This is when the muscle is typically in its shortened position or mid-range, and the contraction happens statically, meaning the muscle neither shortens nor lengthens. Think about feeling your bicep when giving the double 'gun show'. You have your elbow flexed, squeeze your bicep and feel the contraction at its strongest in the static position once the elbow is flexed – that's an isometric contraction. Physiotherapists often use isometrics during early-stage rehabilitation with injured muscle groups as a way of re-activating those muscles before strengthening them. We're about to do the same for your diaphragm.

EXERCISE: BLOCKED INHALE

When using this as an activation exercise rather than the assessment, start by shaking out and relaxing your neck, chest and shoulders. Then:

- Locate the centre point of your central diaphragm tendon just below your sternum (breastplate), an inch or so down between where your two lower ribs angle away diagonally from your sternum.
- Rub that area a bit to send some sensory input to your brain, signalling that you want this area to initiate the movement of inhalation instead of your chest, neck or shoulders.
- I like to keep a finger on that area, where the isometric contraction – which feels like a pulse – will come from.
- Take a normal breath in and out so that the next thing your respiratory centre wants to do is to breathe in.

- Pinch your nose and hold your breath; try to breathe in but keep holding your breath so that no air can come in. You should feel a 'pulse' or contraction of the diaphragm.
- When you relax and stop trying to breathe, the contraction or pulse stops.
- Try one or two contractions at a time and then relax.

As you are holding your breath and not letting any air in, the diaphragm can't move, so instead of moving down and flattening out as it would normally, it pulses (isometric contraction). You might feel like it is popping out of your stomach, underneath where your finger is below your sternum. Repeat this a couple of times until you feel very connected to your diaphragm and can activate it at will.

It could take a few days of practice, but there will be a light-bulb moment where you'll finally feel what a decent diaphragm contraction feels like, and it will be a game changer!

Exercise: Supine diaphragmatic breathing mechanics

Now we can activate our diaphragm, it's time to start feeling it moving as we practise the skill of diaphragmatic breathing mechanics. As we know, diaphragmatic breathing helps increase tidal volume and regulate breathing rate when running.

The position of our ribcage dictates the function of the diaphragm, so we want our ribcage and pelvis in good alignment. The ribcage and pelvis have a very important relationship with each other, and they mirror one another. If the ribs project upwards, the pelvis goes down; if the pelvis rolls forwards, the ribs tilt up. So, we'll be using the semi-supine position we mentioned previously to get started with this exercise.

EXERCISE: SUPINE DIAPHRAGMATIC BREATHING MECHANICS

A full video tutorial of the following exercise can be found online at www.thebreathrunningcoach.com/breathing-mechanics

- Lie down on the floor in the semi-supine position.
- Create a long spine and space between the bottom of your ribcage and your pelvis and relax your stomach.
- Create some gentle suction with your tongue so that it's placed at the roof of the mouth, then close your mouth.
- Look slightly behind you, rather than straight up, so your chin lifts about 1–2cm, opening your airway. It should feel like your pallet is stacked on top of your throat.
- Rather than breathing up your nose, breathe into your face, so you sense the air flowing back through the nostrils towards the back of your throat.
- As you breathe very quietly, ideally silently (remember, quiet breathing prevents over-breathing at rest), place your hands so your palms are on the outside of the lowest ribs and your fingertips in the middle just above your belly button.
- As you inhale, keep it as slow and quiet as possible, but see how much air you can get into your lungs when you fill them from the bottom up, expanding the ribcage all around you, with the diaphragm initiating the inhale.
- With practice (remember, breathing is a skill you can improve) you should be able to feel the inhale being 360 degrees in nature.
- On the exhale, keep the breath quiet, ideally silent, feel the ribs under your palms move back down and in, and the diaphragm moving back up to its resting position.

We are trying to increase the tidal volume as much as possible, but the speed or rate of breathing should be as slow as possible so that we practise taking the diaphragm through its complete range of motion (ZOA) without over-breathing.

Keeping it quiet and very slow is important while practising at rest, but it might be a little challenging at first. If it is, you know you are creating some form of adaptation. It's a good thing when the body notices something is different – it naturally wants to do what it has always done, but this means it's learning ... we're getting better at breathing!

Key external and internal sensations

External sensation:

- As you breathe in through your nose, feel your ribs move up and out laterally underneath your hands.
- A helpful visualisation for the movement of the ribs is like two bucket handles, one for each side of the ribcage. Split your ribcage in your mind into two halves. The bucket handle on each side pivots about the sternum at the front of you and the thoracic spine at the back. As you inhale, imagine the bucket handle moving up on either side of you.

Internal sensation:

- As you breathe in, feel your diaphragm moving down towards your pelvis like a pump on the inside. You can't feel this with your hands, as the diaphragm is a deep tissue, so you need to sense this internally. You should feel the pressure you create in the abdomen. This creates the intra-abdominal pressure that causes your abdominal region to expand as the diaphragm draws down and flattens when it contracts on the inhale.

- If you find it hard to feel the diaphragm, do a couple of blocked inhalations to activate it so you can feel it contract more strongly, and then repeat the last step.

Progression with 'breath control': Slow exhale and pause

Once you've got the hang of the optimal breathing mechanics semi-supine on the floor, we can start to make it more challenging with breath control.

Remember, carbon dioxide is a key player in our ventilation drive (desire to inhale), and we want to 'make friends' with it. We are going to practise slowing down our breathing so much that we feel slightly out of breath. When we exhale slower than our body naturally wants to, it means carbon dioxide isn't leaving the body as fast. Our central chemoreceptors in the brain stem notice this and our urge to breathe will be stronger. As that urge increases, our auto setting of wanting to get air in quickly means we'd normally then rush the inhale, and the increased speed of the inhale means it will come fast and shallow from the chest and not the diaphragm. But in this exercise, you know it's coming, as it's not a surprise, and so you're going to practise softening that urge and controlling your breathing with the power of your diaphragm.

EXERCISE: PROGRESSION WITH 'BREATH CONTROL'

- Lie on the floor in the same semi-supine position as before.
- Perform the same steps to take a full inhale.
- Gradually start to slow down your exhale as much as you can, to the point that you make yourself feel a little out of breath, but not so much that you can't control the next inhale.
- When the urge to inhale increases, choose to still use the diaphragm rather than the chest first; choose to keep it quiet and slow.
- I like to push in on the ribs with the palms a little bit so that I can feel some slight resistance from my hands, which the ribs and diaphragm have to overcome – this helps with the breath control.

- As you get better with your breath control and improve your carbon dioxide tolerance, you can progress to adding some pauses at the end of the slower, extended exhale.
- As you pause at the end of the exhale, carbon dioxide will accumulate in the lungs and blood to a greater degree, so your urge to inhale will become stronger and it will be a little more challenging to control that breath.

It's a bit like when you are running at a faster pace than you're used to: your legs are working harder, and your lungs and blood are accumulating more carbon dioxide. You'll want to breathe harder and faster, resulting in more-inefficient chest breathing. But if you can control the rate and urge to breathe, as we are practising here, you have more control to mechanically ventilate efficiently, more like the elites!

Exercise: Exhale bridge – repositioning ribcage

I first came across this exercise from Dana Santas, during a podcast interview I had with her. She's a mobility, breathing and mind–body coach, working with professional athletes in American sports like the NHL and NFL. She explained that all too often she sees poor exhalation in athletes because they can't get their ribs down and in. Why is exhaling important when we all focus on getting the air in? Well, as Dana said: 'If the ribs can't come down and in (flexion and internal rotation) they stay widened, which means the diaphragm is in a flatter position and can't get back to its resting state.'

I then came across a variation of this exhale bridge during a workshop series with Dr Cobb from Z Health Performance and I remember thinking, *this is exactly the same thing that Dana Santas was talking about*. When I see two highly trained educational experts in my field, both working with elite and Olympic athletes, saying the same thing, it's a potential game changer – and that's exactly what the exhale bridge is!

Before I take you through the steps of this exercise, it's important to know why we are doing it in this specific position. When we do an active exhale (like when running), we are trying to get the air out on the exhale a little faster than at rest when the exhale can be passive. When the exhale is active, we use our skeletal muscles, namely our abdominal muscles and obliques, to force the air out more strongly. Try this: put your hands on your rectus abdominis, your six-pack muscles (they are there somewhere, I promise) and do a really strong exhale out of your mouth – what do you feel? Your abs tense like mad, right? You probably brought your sternum down and flexed your spine.

Our rectus abdominis are typically strong (relative to other core musculature), and we are used to having a flexed spine from too much sitting, etc. Your ribs don't have to move downwards and inwards much if you just flex your spine and compress the whole ribcage down during an exhale. The ribs, however, are supposed to move downwards and inwards on the exhale, as Dana Santas explained. If your ribs are restricted and your obliques weak, rather than the ribs moving inwards and downwards, we still exhale and expel the air, but it's by compensating with spinal flexion. Spinal flexion is a more global movement, using bigger muscles and more energy, which is, therefore, less efficient. What does that do to your tall posture necessary for good running form? You effectively shrink when you flex the spine!

Hence why we do this exercise in a low floor bridge position, to stop any spinal flexion compensation. You simply can't flex your spine in a low floor bridge. If during your ribcage assessments, you noticed your infra-sternal angle was wider than 90 degrees and/or your lower back was arched with your ribcage pushed forwards, then you'll notice big improvements with this exercise. If your hip flexors and hamstrings are especially tight, you'll also notice improvements in your hips. So, it's always good to do a little test and retest, before and after a few reps. Something as simple as trying to touch your toes before and after is ideal.

EXERCISE: EXHALE BRIDGE

A full video tutorial of the following exercise can be found online at www.thebreathrunningcoach.com/exhale-bridge

a)

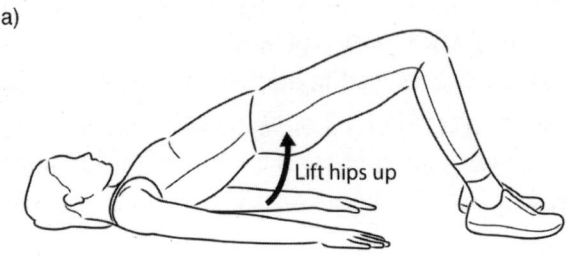

Lift hips up

b)

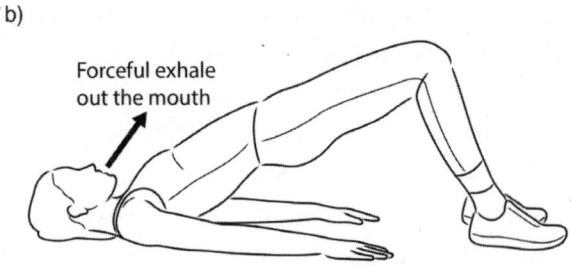

Forceful exhale out the mouth

Maximise your exhale, and your six pack, with the exhale floor bridge!

The emphasis of this exercise is all about the exhalation to get the ribs down and in.

- From the semi-supine position, engage your glutes and push through your feet to raise your hips up into a low floor bridge position so that your hips are just 3–4 inches off the ground.

- Take a normal inhale through your nose, but then use your mouth to allow a more forceful exhale. Forcefully drive all of the air out of your lungs. Feel your abs and obliques tense as the ribs move downwards and inwards – it's like the ultimate six-pack exercise: welcome to six-pack city!
- Once it feels like all the air is out, pause and hold your breath with empty lungs.
- While pausing (still holding your breath on empty lungs), your job is to pull your bum and ribcage down to the floor together. You should feel that the whole of your ribcage is pushed into the floor underneath you, as well as your bum. (The main mistake people make is only bringing their bum to the floor and leaving the ribs sticking up and arching their back.)
- In this position, you are in optimal alignment with your ribcage and pelvis at the end of an exhalation where your ribs have moved beautifully downwards and inwards. The perfect position of a complete exhalation – the perfect starting point for the most optimally mechanical inhalation. Remember: a good inhale starts with a good exhale.
- As you've paused and held your breath on empty lungs while repositioning the ribcage with the pelvis, you'll have a slightly stronger urge to inhale than normal.
- Breathe in quietly and controlled, as you learned in the exercise on page 153, filling from the bottom up, 360-degree expansion and initiated from the diaphragm.
- Relax after the inhale and calm your breathing through your nose, taking a short break to reset.
- Perform three to five strong exhales like this, resetting between each rep. This is a great 'activation' exercise to use in warm-ups before running and training sessions.

PROGRESSION: EXHALE BRIDGE WITH ARMS OVERHEAD

A lovely progression for this exercise for runners, especially those prone to rib flaring and extended positions when running (back arched and pelvis rolled forward – anterior pelvic tilt), is performing the exercise with the arms overhead. To do this, follow all the same steps, except when you lift your bum up off the floor at the start, also lift your arms up over your head, elbows as straight as possible and hands on the floor. Keep your hands overhead, touching the floor for the rest of the exercise – it can be helpful to 'trap' them under something like your sofa or hold on to something to keep them fixed. When you pull your ribcage and bum to the floor after exhaling all the air out of your lungs, it will be challenging to get your ribcage to the floor, especially if your thoracic spine is tight. But this arm position helps to get your ribcage in a better position, and opens up your thoracic spine, which are two keys to unlocking the power of your diaphragm and taller running posture. Improving not just your breathing but your running form too – making you a stronger runner.

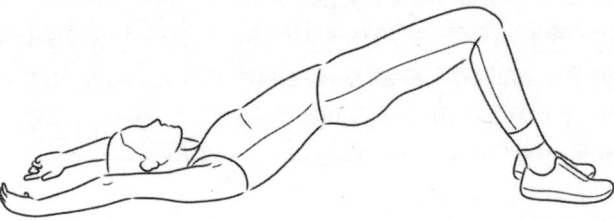

Challenge your ribcage position with this progression with arms overhead

We can all benefit

Who could benefit most from improving diaphragmatic breathing? Performance physiotherapist Gemma Jefferson, who works with elite, Paralympic and Olympic athletes, said, 'There isn't a single athlete I've worked with that when I've treated them, couldn't make improvements to their breathing mechanics.' The improvement you feel in your running might come sooner than you think.

As it did with Marc, a keen runner trying to get under the three-hour mark in his marathon and under 35 minutes for his 10km. After working on his ribcage positioning, activating his diaphragm and practising some diaphragmatic breathing mechanics, he made huge improvements. We retested a hill run and he unleashed the power of his diaphragm. He ran at a faster pace, yet felt more relaxed and in control with a lower heart rate.

Despite running slightly faster, by using his diaphragm to help control the rate and size of his breaths, he ran stronger and it felt easier – and that was in just one session!

A few months later, with a lot of training, he ran 2:57 at Barcelona marathon.

Biggest mistake: Belly breathing

One of the biggest mistakes we see with diaphragmatic breathing is oversimplifying it to 'belly breathing'. Anatomically, we've highlighted that the diaphragm itself is not in your stomach or belly and neither are your lungs, of course. Yes, you feel the 'belly' move as you create intra-abdominal pressure with diaphragmatic breathing, which we'll learn in the next chapter is vital to improving hip mobility and reducing hip pain. But your belly just moving out is a one-dimensional mistake.

As common as the term belly breathing is – and with good reason because it takes the attention away from the upper chest-dominant breathing – it's a little one-dimensional. You can move your belly up towards the ceiling while lying down and practising belly breathing, but without the lateral and posterior expansion of the ribcage. With belly breathing it's too easy to miss the important movement up and out of the ribcage.

Lying down on a yoga mat doing some gentle relaxation breathing with only the belly moving is fine, but it's not the full story of optimal diaphragmatic breathing mechanics. If the ribs don't move, the diaphragm doesn't function fully. And if the ribs don't move, the spine can't move and you end up with a stiff thoracic spine which affects our tall running posture. Imagine a balloon blowing up. It's not just the front of the balloon that expands out, the balloon expands 360 degrees in all directions. Just your belly moving out when you're running is perhaps an improvement from pumping your upper chest, but you are missing out on the full power of your diaphragm if the ribcage and the ribs themselves are not moving in synchronisation with the diaphragm. We want to unleash the full power of our diaphragm; your ribs moving in synchronisation with the diaphragm allows you to feel its full superpowers!

Small changes create big improvements

Getting better at diaphragmatic breathing is about getting started. One of the most important things is being aware of how you are currently breathing. It always starts with awareness. If you're not aware of it, then you can't do anything about changing it. You can start building awareness right now by asking yourself the question 'can I feel my diaphragm moving?' as you breathe. Being aware of breathing at rest is often easier than during the challenge of running, so is a great place to start. If you're unsure or don't feel your diaphragm, use the DAT (see page 126) to activate your diaphragm and really feel it engage. Remember, you have specific mechanoreceptors in the lung wall, diaphragm and ribcage, and we just need to know how to use them.

The exercises outlined in this chapter are performed lying down to make it easy for you to get started and get a feel for how the ribs and diaphragm are supposed to move together. Practise these a few times a week, and if you can get into the habit of doing them before you warm-up for a run, even better. When practising, start to link together other things we've learned, as stacking all the little tips and techniques together really starts to add up. For example, your tongue position and airway that you learned about in chapter 6 really helps your diaphragmatic breathing. Linking your diaphragmatic breathing and tongue posture helps with your nasal breathing during low-intensity runs. Start adding up all the one percenters and you begin to see transformations in your running.

The good news is we have even more one percenters coming up in the next chapter.

We said we'd make friends with possibly the most important muscle in your body and certainly the most important muscle for breathing. Now you understand where your diaphragm is, and its relationship with the ribcage. You have simple tools to make friends with it, learn how it feels to use it optimally and practise the skill of diaphragmatic breathing mechanics.

Like any skill, it takes some time to master. Eventually, though, it becomes the new 'auto' – and one that's optimal, not a compensation. Your new automatic breathing will be more efficient, use less energy and help you stay relaxed, making you, ultimately, a stronger runner.

> **Key takeaways**
>
> - The diaphragm has multiple roles to play – the most important for runners are its roles in ventilation, creating postural stability and improving force transfer.
> - The alignment of the ribcage and pelvis is key to the optimal function of the diaphragm and increasing your ZOA (zone of apposition).
> - Breathing is a skill and with practice you improve your mechanical ventilation through the use of your diaphragm and articulation of your ribs like bucket handles.
> - Exhales are just as important as inhales. Getting the ribs down and in with an exhale allows for the correct starting point of the diaphragm for the next inhale.

Working with Jacko on nasal-only breathing was a game changer in my journey to running a sub-3-hour marathon in Barcelona. Through his expert coaching, I learned how to slow my breath, stay calm under pressure, and breathe using the power of my diaphragm in a much more controlled and efficient way.

Honestly, I never thought something as simple as breathing could have such a big impact, but it really has.

Marc Swinbank, marathon PB now 2:57

CHAPTER 9

More mobility and less pain

Transforming your running with breathing isn't just about using the power of your diaphragm to get more air in and out, it can unlock your hips and spine, potentially reducing stiffness and pain as you melt into a flow state with synchronisation between your running and breathing.

Breathing connects everything

Lying on the physio's couch with the therapist messing around with my stomach and the bottom of my ribcage felt particularly unpleasant, and not just because I was seeing her because of a shoulder injury. 'Oh wow, your diaphragm is really tight,' explained Kim, as she prodded and probed my abdomen. I wanted to make all sorts of noises, the pain from the tightness made me feel sick. I managed to blurt out something along the lines of, 'I don't really care, Kim, it's my shoulder I've hurt!'

Kim was aware of an important kinetic chain link that the ribcage and diaphragm have through the whole of the human body, which back in 2015, I was completely oblivious to. Kim was so nice that reading the tone in my voice, knowing I wasn't ready to make the link between the diaphragm and my shoulder, she changed tactics and moved upstream. As she did some more traditional release work on my shoulder, she tried to subtly and gently to open up my mind to the possibility that my tight diaphragm could be causing me some issues elsewhere in the kinetic chain. I was working as a strength and conditioning coach with Paralympic athletes at the time and, although kinetic chain principles were something we understood as strength coaches, the role of the diaphragm was never spoken about. I didn't have any appreciation or education in it, and I just wasn't ready to hear it. But a seed had been planted, which was slowly growing in the background, unbeknown to me.

Increasing stability and reducing pain through breathing

We're going to look at how our breathing influences how the body moves, not just for the act of breathing but for running itself. We'll see how we can reduce stiffness and pain, improve mobility of the hips, shoulders and spine, with the link being our diaphragm and how it provides much needed stability.

There has been more research into the multifunctional component of the diaphragm, not just as a breathing muscle but as a postural stabiliser. The cascading positive or negative effects on the rest of the movement, stability and mobility within the body as a result of either good or bad function of the diaphragm. In 2001 one study highlighted the significance of the diaphragm in postural stabilisation, which gets challenged and even reduced as our breathing demand increases.[1]

Ten years later, studies have linked abnormal function of the diaphragm to things such as lower back pain.[2] A link was discovered in 2014 about its ability to improve Functional Movement Screen scores, noting a link between breathing and improved movement, stability and mobility.[3] That was something I've encountered with all the top physiotherapists I've worked with in elite sports.

I was introduced to Bob Stewart, the Medical Lead for England Rugby Senior Men's Team, as we were both visiting one of the England players who was rehabbing an injury. We hit it off straight away due to a joint passion for the benefits of breathing for the players. Bob is a tremendous physiotherapist who cares deeply about the players, and you can see it in his work. He explained, 'I was mainly looking to help down-regulate players as an adjunct to our recovery protocols. Cognitive stress is generally high for most athletes in international camps from both a performance demand and learning perspective so as a performance team we felt this was a key area for us to develop.' He added that this then piqued his interest 'in the biomechanical and neurological benefits of breathing. Having gone and undertaken some courses and read some books (including the *Oxygen Advantage*), I found that I could have a bigger impact on musculoskeletal health and movement efficiency through breathing than I could at times with my manual skills.'

Top athletes across many sports and the medical staff who support them are starting to use the benefits of breathing increasingly within their training and rehabilitation programmes. I've personally witnessed it within England Rugby Union (men's and women's teams), England Women's football, British Cycling (BMX), MMA as well as within athletics.

Specifically, for runners, the relationship between the diaphragm and pelvis is a key one because so many of us have tight hips. Those of us who are longer-distance runners, especially in the 'ultra' world, running 100km or more, it's fair to say it's more like a shuffle than running. The tight hips are often attributed to all of the running and the gait being small and repetitive. I'm the oldest I've ever been (43 as I write this book), doing the most running I've ever done in my life, yet my hips are the most flexible (when I get things right), which doesn't add up. It wasn't always the case. When I was a poor breather, not only were my hips tight after long runs, but my back, neck and shoulders would be tight too! What changed? My breathing, and it affected the rest of my body and my running.

The stiffness we feel in other parts of our body can also be affected by the way we breathe when running. This relationship between your breathing cycle and your running cycle is known in the literature as Locomotor-Respiratory Coupling (LRC). There are two distinct phases in running and breathing. In running, first when your foot strikes the ground and you experience ground reaction forces, and then when you are flying in the air and nothing is touching the ground. In breathing, you have inhalation and increased stability in your trunk (when breathing skilfully with your diaphragm), and then when exhaling and air is leaving your lungs, you reduce dynamic stabilisation internally from reduced pressure.

When the end of your exhale is constantly linked with a foot strike on the same leg, it can lead to more stiffness and pain somewhere on that side, as you're less stable at the end of an exhale. It's even been linked to stitches, for those who suffer with them. The good news is we're going to learn how to effectively synchronise the right parts of our breathing cycle with our foot strikes to reduce pain and stiffness, as well as enhance the efficiency of our breathing and running economy.

A canister of pressure in your core

Firstly, we're going to start with the effect of breathing on our mobility and a particularly problematic area of running – our hips and the negative effect on our stride length.

I spoke again to performance physiotherapist Gemma Jefferson about the correlation between tight hips and breathing mechanics. She described to me that, time and time again, when treating athletes complaining of tight hips and hip pain, if she identified that they also had dysfunctional breathing (particularly overuse of upper chest accessory breathing muscles), the hip tightness and pain wouldn't go away until she restored diaphragmatic breathing; it wasn't just a matter of treating 'tight hip flexors'.

So, what was the root cause and how was breathing an integral part of the solution?

Something she observed was a correlation between runners with highly toned abdominals and a lack of diaphragmatic breathing. She explained for example, 'a female athlete with six-pack abs to die for. Even at rest just standing talking the abs are popping out at you, you could have drawn them on. If you have that much tone around your stomach at rest, it's just going to be harder to expand the lower ribcage and diaphragmatically breathe. If we then restrict the lower ribcage with tone and tension around our abdominals, then the upper ribcage will "naturally" have to move instead.'

Gemma uses an analogy of a canister, where the top of the canister is the diaphragm, the pelvic floor is the bottom, and the sides are the obliques and paraspinals, with the transverse abdominis at the front. She explained that the pressure needs to be maintained when transferring force, like when your foot hits the ground in running. Gemma explained: 'If there isn't enough pressure in that system, like a coke can it can be easily squashed, deformed and rotated. When a coke can is open and you've lost the pressure, you can squash it. That can be your foot hitting the floor when you are running, you will collapse, you lose force and you're not going to be able to produce the same ground reaction force you need.'

With upper chest breathing, it's like opening that canister and losing pressure out of the system. Gemma explained, 'If you don't have that pressure in the canister, you will find stability elsewhere. Typically, we see hip flexors picking up the slack. So hip flexors get tight and we lose hip extension which reduces stride length. Then you're not using your glutes, you probably can't fire into your hamstrings, you're not pushing through your big toe – it's crazy what you lose when you think about it.'

Finally, Gemma explained how she uses diaphragmatic breathing with athletes to help release those tight hips: 'I've got three athletes currently that before big races in the call room (warm-up, pre-race) all have breathing exercises to do, because it will improve their hip range of motion.' She goes as far to say that she is 'convinced poor breathing mechanics are related to a lot of injuries, not traumatic or impact injuries but things like stiff hips, lower back pain, sore Achilles – if we scanned them it wouldn't show much other than a little inflammation. The solution is we need to teach the brain to believe the stability is going to be coming from somewhere else – the pressure in the canister. Our motor control has to know you are stable enough that you don't need to compensate with the hip flexors tightening back up.' And it's good breathing mechanics at the heart of that solution.

Locomotor-respiratory coupling (LRC)

I'm sure if you've done enough running, like me you've experienced some foot, knee, hip or Achilles pain, or maybe all of the above! Like me, I'm sure you never thought it could be caused by your breathing, let alone the pain being relieved by breathing. I had some ongoing foot and heel pain – let's call it undiagnosed plantar fasciitis – which led me to discover the second link breathing has in relation to pain when running, and finally heal my heel pain!

It was the type of pain that didn't stop me running most of the time. It was just uncomfortable, very annoying and lasted about two years until I understood this link between my breathing cycle and my foot strikes. It was only ever on the left foot. I must have been doing something different on the left than the right. It turns out I was.

LRC links your movement (locomotion) with your breathing (respiration), with some fascinating research into it. Two things jumped out at me immediately. Firstly, it's another thing elite runners naturally do – they sync their breathing with their cadence, often unconsciously.[4] Anything the elites are doing, and especially naturally rather than specifically training, is something I always pay attention to. Secondly, it's common to develop a pattern of running and breathing that results in landing repeatedly on the same foot at the end of each exhale.

A 2022 review article explained how repeated landing on the same foot strike on exhalation can result in abdominal pain and a stitch, as well as things like the foot pain I was experiencing.[5] Digging a little deeper, it appeared the impact on the body and your foot is different on an inhale than on an exhale, especially at the end of the exhale when the lungs are relatively empty. Similar to Gemma Jefferson's coke can analogy – an empty coke can is easily crushed when the canister doesn't have pressure in it. You have the least internal pressure at the end of the exhale. It makes sense, then, at the end of the exhale, the forces coming back from the ground as your foot strikes (ground reaction force) could cause you, as in the case of my foot, some issues if the end of the exhale always happens on the same foot.

I was keen to find out if I always landed on my left foot at the end of my exhales. I went out for a little 5km at a steady, comfortable pace. I settled into my running first before my observational experiment took place. I started to be aware of how many steps I took on my inhale and how many steps I took on my exhale. Inhale one, two, three, four as I counted four foot strikes. Exhale one, two, three, four as I counted four foot strikes. Four steps in and four steps out seemed to feel comfortable and relaxed. *Good news*, I thought, *eight is a nice even number, so I must be taking the same number of strides with each foot. I'm like the elite runners, naturally gifted to alternate foot strikes.* I then started to notice my foot hitting the floor at the end of the exhale, when the canister was almost empty. As I counted my exhales, one, two, three and then the fourth final step, my left foot hit the floor. *Well, I've got eight strides to the next end of exhale foot strike, so that's fine*, I thought, which would then be my right foot. The next exhale was coming and again I counted one, two, three and then the fourth strike – and my left foot hit the floor again. How could it be my left foot again?

I counted my four steps on the inhale and four on the exhale for the next few breathing cycles, and sure enough it was my left. The inhale then started with a right foot, followed by left, then right and left again for those four steps of the inhale. Then the exhale started with a right foot strike, then left, then right and the fourth foot strike was back on the left foot. This left me in a predicament. Either I couldn't count or didn't know my right from my left. Neither was correct. I was doing eight strides, four on the inhale and four on the exhale and that even number of total steps was exactly why I was hitting the floor at the end of the exhale always with my left foot. Was it coincidence? Was it really the reason for my sore foot, heel and Achilles? My pain could be coming from an old injury or something else. Initially I brushed it off. I didn't like counting my steps and I didn't like being wrong.

The next few days when running I'd try to forget about it, but every now and again, I'd just check how many strides I was taking and which foot was striking the floor at the end of the exhale. You guessed it, it was my left foot.

I couldn't hide or deny it. The natural rhythm that I liked had me landing on my left side over and over again at the end of the exhale. Would evening that out be the key to finally healing my sore foot and heel? There was only one way to find out. I started using a four-step inhale and a five-step exhale, and not only in just over a week or so did my foot and heel pain go away, I found the foot counting and sequencing almost hypnotising. I'd be bobbing along, counting my steps, feeling quite happy with myself when every other exhale the foot would swap like magic. It got to the point where I was just in a rhythm and I didn't even have to count four steps on the inhale. I knew what it felt like in terms of duration and ribcage expansion, and then I'd naturally just exhale until the correct foot hit the ground last, swapping each time. Time just melted away and I'd run for an hour and it would feel like 10 minutes. When running up a steep climb or mountain, rather than wondering how much further it was, I was just counting my steps and, all of a sudden, I was at the top. Not only at the top easier, also feeling less out of breath.

Why did I feel less out of breath? What else was this LRC doing?

Excited and intrigued, I discovered more research than I was expecting. Some of its origins seem to date back to the 1980s. It's something that Dr Jack Daniels, who's been called 'the world's best running coach', covers in his book *Daniels' Running Formula*.[6] The more recent literature suggests it's 'likely modulated by an interaction of mechanical, neurological, and metabolic interactions during running', with a direct link in humans 'between the respiratory and locomotor central pattern generators in the spinal cord. Suggesting LRC is a result of the "minimal effort" hypothesis of breathing'.[7] It can potentially make breathing easier by reducing the workload of the breathing muscles, creating a rhythm that allows easier access to flow state and relaxation.

How does syncing your breathing with your steps make any difference to how hard your breathing muscles have to work? You might wonder, as I did. The studies in that review paper explain that when your foot hits the ground, depending on where you are in your breathing cycle, it can have an effect on your tidal volume, affecting overall ventilation by over 10%.[8] 'This could be detrimental when the timing of foot strike is out of phase (unsynchronized) with breath onset (flow reversal; FR) but additive when in-phase (synchronized). When the inhale is synchronized with peak visceral downward velocity, it pulls on the diaphragm, increasing the velocity of shortening.'[9]

This means when the start of the inhale is in time with when your foot strikes the floor, the ground reaction force on your body actually helps with the downward contraction phase of the diaphragm. As you inhale, the diaphragm wants to move down and then the force pulling down on your trunk, as your foot hits the floor, makes it easier for your diaphragm to function. Pretty cool, really!

The researchers noted the piston-style movement of the trunk due to gravity and ground reaction force combined with the rhythmic arm action had a 'substantial effect' and that 'LRC has a physiologically significant mechanical effect on breathing dynamics'.[10] All of which effectively leads to what the researchers describe as 'passive assistance' during running and breathing. This helps to increase total ventilation without increasing the metabolic work of the breathing muscles – ultimately increasing the efficiency of breathing and leading to improved running economy and performance.[11]

It's not only the synchronisation that helps reduce the effort of the inhale – it's the exhales too. I noted pain relief with my foot and ankle when I was not always landing on the same foot at the end of my exhales, but there's more. The researchers state that the 'active exhales may further enhance the exhale phase in combination with LRC, as concentric contraction of the abdominal and pelvic floor musculature may optimize visceral compressive forces when synchronized with step-driven flows . . . it may contribute to a delayed onset of ventilatory muscle fatigue, especially at high exercise intensities, long exercise durations.'[12]

This means when we are in synchronisation, we not only match our inhales with our foot strike to reduce the effort of the diaphragm – and increase ventilation at less energy cost – but we also improve the exhale phase by synchronising the foot strike with the exhale too. This takes advantage of the exhalation muscular contraction to both stabilise the trunk and force the air out of the lungs, which can lead to less respiratory muscle fatigue and improved running economy.

Finally, combining the benefits of syncing your breathing with your foot strike also appears to modulate our all-important breathing rate. It allows for an increased tidal volume at no extra energy cost, helping freely increase total ventilation by over 10%. Breathing is essentially easier and also slower, meaning it's more efficient, which allows us to relax and find our flow. Studies have noted that direct feedback from the foot strike and being immersed in that experience can lead us into a flow state more easily.[13]

Since trying out LRC to help relieve my foot pain, I certainly noticed the rhymical nature of LRC that researchers described as 'comforting, sedating and hypnotic'.[14] I experienced greater relaxation and a loss of the sense of time. I was in flow state and my breathing helped me access it.

TRY THIS

Synchronising breath with steps

The practical element of starting to use LRC with the different ratios I've developed for different paced runs is detailed in chapter 13. For now, what I want you to test is how does it feel to try to count your steps while being aware of your breathing. Notice if you like it or if it puts you off.

- How many steps do you take during your inhale?
- How many steps on your exhale?
- At the end of the exhales, are you always landing on the same foot?

Have a play with what it feels like to change how many steps you take for an inhale and for an exhale. Experiment with it playfully, initially, to get a taste for it. I hated it at first but now it's my go-to tool for finding flow state. Just be inquisitive to start with and get some practice before I give you some specific ratios for different gears to use in chapter 13.

Breathing mobilisations

The other practical exercise for this chapter is going to focus on the breathing mobilisations to help open up the ribcage itself, release the diaphragm and the spine and hips. Olympic 400m runner Iwan Thomas explained that he used to get massage release on his diaphragm from his physiotherapist and always felt like it was easier to breathe and could take a larger inhale after the treatment. These breathing mobilisations are going to help release your diaphragm and mobilise the ribcage to the same effect, but are simple for you to do on your own at home.

Coaches and educators who have been very helpful in developing these have been Dr Cobb, Dana Santas and author of *Body by Breath* Jill Miller, who all have unique ways of using breathing to optimise movement and mobility. I've taken elements from what each of them has taught me over the years and developed what's most effective for the athletes and runners I personally work with.

Test and retest mobility

Make sure you use the movement assessments from chapter 7 before and after these breathing mobilisation drills to ensure you notice the difference in your hips and spine. If you check before and after each separate drill, it helps you to understand which mobilisation specifically is best for your body. I've chosen three that have had a positive response from all athletes regardless of the individualised approach some athletes need. These three cover the back, sides and front of the ribcage.

A key principle we'll follow with each mobilisation is moving the ribs from the inside out with our breathing. We'll be positioning the body to restrict one area so we specifically target another area of the ribcage to open up.

Exercise: Back of ribcage – Kneeling posterior mobilisation

This is one of my favourite mobilisations to teach because it's so simple, yet the effects are so dramatic. It's something I've worked on with many professional and international rugby players, particularly due to the nature of a contact sport on the thoracic region. Navdeep Singh Sandhu, lead physiotherapist at Sale Sharks, who's worked with the England rugby team, explained, 'With the thoracic spine it's an area that in general we just don't train well and therefore have lots of issues with it. The breathing mobilisations you've taught the players have been a game changer.' Check your thoracic spine rotation before and after this mobilisation and be prepared for some game-changing mobility, which can transform your tall, efficient running posture.

EXERCISE: BACK OF RIBCAGE

A full video tutorial of the following exercise can be found online at www.thebreathrunningcoach.com/back-mobilisation

- Kneel on the floor on all fours.
- Have your hips stacked vertically on top of your knees and your shoulders vertically stacked on top of your elbows, with forearms and palms facing down on the floor.
- Tuck your pelvis in, hump your back up towards the ceiling, and tense your abs to restrict the front of the ribcage so the back will have to open up.
- Push your elbows into the ground to protract your shoulder blades around your ribcage and lean slightly forward so there is a tiny bit more force through your shoulders.
- Inhale as hard as possible through your nose, feeling the space between your shoulder blades expand and stretch.
- Pause at the top of that inhale for a second or two to feel the stretch.
- Let a bit of air out without losing the stretch so you can take another big breath in, 'stacking' another inhale on top.
- Again, pause at the top to feel a bigger stretch and repeat so that you've stacked three inhales on top of each other.

- At the top of the third inhale, suck in a bit of extra air through the mouth. The more air you can pack in on the inside, the more the ribs will move out at the back.
- Pause and feel the strongest stretch between your shoulder blades and relax as you control your exhale out of the nose.

Try to control the air leaving your nose rather than letting it just fall out of your mouth in a big sigh at the end. Practising the skill of controlling your exhale will come in handy when we talk about recovery in chapter 12, so you can get a head start by creating good habits now.

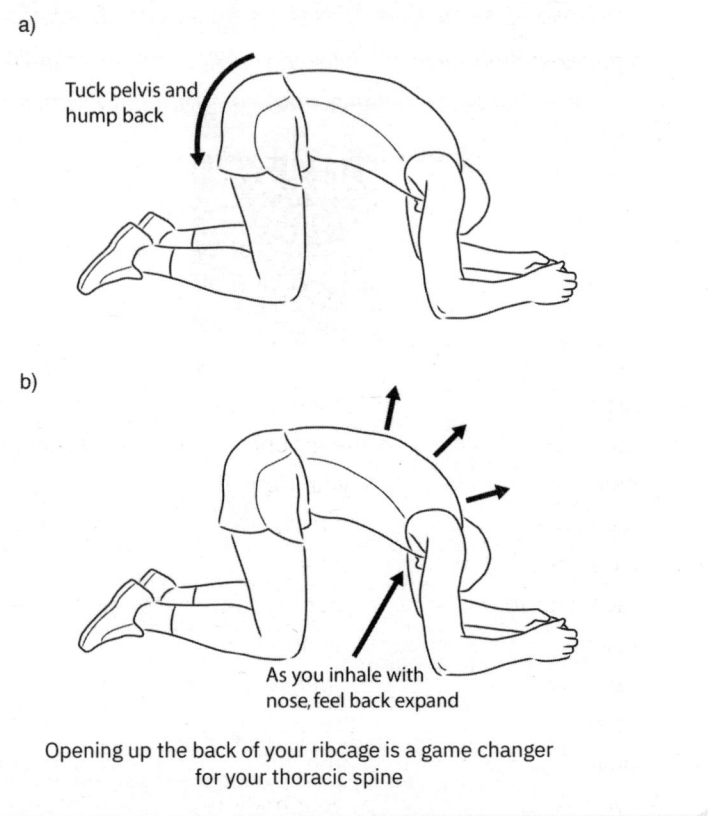

Opening up the back of your ribcage is a game changer for your thoracic spine

Have a little break for a few seconds because this isn't passive stretching. If you did it right, you'll know what I mean when I say it's active; you are working hard to create that expansion. That's one of the reasons it works so well and why it's great as part of your warm-up.

Perform this twice and retest your thoracic rotation; even your shoulders and hips may have improved too, so pivotal is the thoracic spine to mobility in the entire body.

Exercise: Side of ribcage – Lunge with reach mobilisation

This mobilisation is great for the hips, as it targets the psoas and quadratus lumborum, so I recommend checking your hip rotation and toe touch before and after this one.

EXERCISE: LUNGE WITH REACH MOBILISATION

A full video tutorial of the following exercise can be found online at www.thebreathrunningcoach.com/side-mobilisation

- Start in a lunge position with your right knee on the floor and left knee up.
- Push back your toes into the ground on the right leg and push your hips forward so you engage your right glute.
- Reach up with your right hand to the ceiling and spread your fingers as wide as possible to torque up the fascia.
- Reach over to the left with your right arm to the point where you get stuck and can't reach over anymore.
- Take a massive inhale with your nose, making the area on the right side expand and stretch. At the top of the inhale, hold your breath for a moment and feel the stretch from the expansion with your breath.
- As you exhale and air leaves your body, relax your right side and allow your ribs on the left to come down, letting yourself now reach further to the left with your right arm.

- In this new position, take another breath and follow the same sequence. Do this three times in a row and then swap sides.

a) Reach up

b) Reach over

Feel expansion as you inhale and hold

Mobilising the side of your ribcage increases your ability to expand it laterally, giving space for your diaphragm

Exercise: Front of ribcage – Exhale floor bridge mobilisation

The front side of your ribcage is targeted not with inhales, like the first two mobilisations, but with exhales. The mobilisation drill is, in fact, one you already know because it's the exhale bridge we did in the last chapter.

When we forcefully and fully exhale in the floor bridge position, the obliques and core have to engage. Not only does this help with ribcage alignment but it actually encourages mobilisation of the ribs themselves to move downwards and inwards effectively. Many of us are tight in the ribs and weak in the obliques and core, so the body compensates by flexing the spine to force the air out as we exhale. The game-changing magic of the exhale bridge is that the bridge position eliminates the compensation of spinal flexion, so you get the mobilisation of the ribs at the front of the body on a full exhale.

EXERCISE: EXHALE FLOOR BRIDGE MOBILISATION

A full video tutorial of the following exercise can be found online at www.thebreathrunningcoach.com/exhale-bridge

The exhale floor bridge can have a really big impact on your hips, so retest your toe touch after doing three of these. If your shoulders and thoracic spine feel particularly tight and you want an extra mobilisation, perform the exhale bridge progression with the arms overhead. Having the hands fixed under something, like your sofa, means when you pull the ribcage down to the floor after the exhale, you get a huge opening of your thoracic spine.

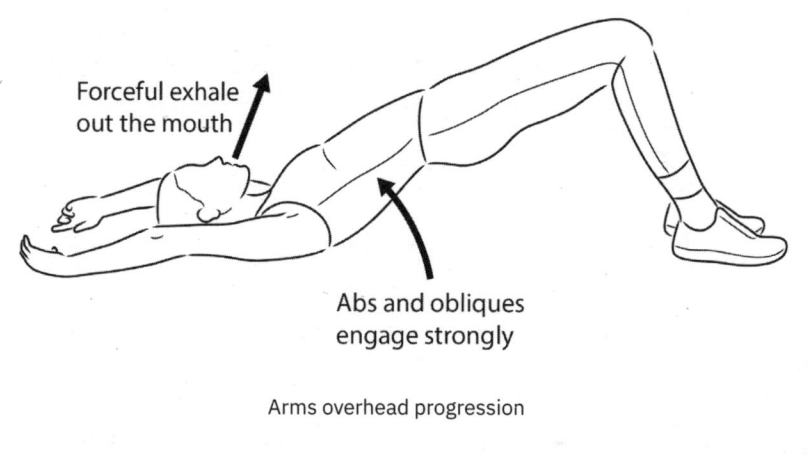

Arms overhead progression

Exercise: Bonus thoracic mobilisation – inhale and exhales combined

The ability for the thoracic region to extend and rotate is key to good running posture and effortless form. Here is a little bonus to combine the inhales and exhales in a rotation pattern. This can be done in any rotational movement, as they all require rotation of the ribcage.

When we rotate to the right, the ribs on the right side of the ribcage move away from the spine, and the ribs on the left move towards the spine. The right-hand ribs move in an inhalation pattern when we rotate to the right, and the ribs on the left move in an exhalation pattern. So, we can use inhales and exhales on each side specifically to target improved rotation of the thoracic spine.

To specifically target the thoracic spine in isolation, I like to use the thoracic rotation assessment position. To make it running specific as part of a warm-up, we can integrate it into a lunge rotation position, for example.

EXERCISE: BONUS THORACIC MOBILISATION

The principle is the same for both:

- Rotate as far as you can to the right in your chosen position.
- When you get stuck and can't rotate any further, hold that position.
- Take a massive forceful inhale through your nose into the right-hand side of your ribcage. Try to expand the right side as much as possible.
- On the exhale, force the air out of pursed lips using the mouth so it is forceful; use the exhale to drive the ribs on the left downwards and inwards.
- Push the ribcage around to the right as the ribs on the left move downwards and inwards.
- Repeat two or three times, and then swap sides.

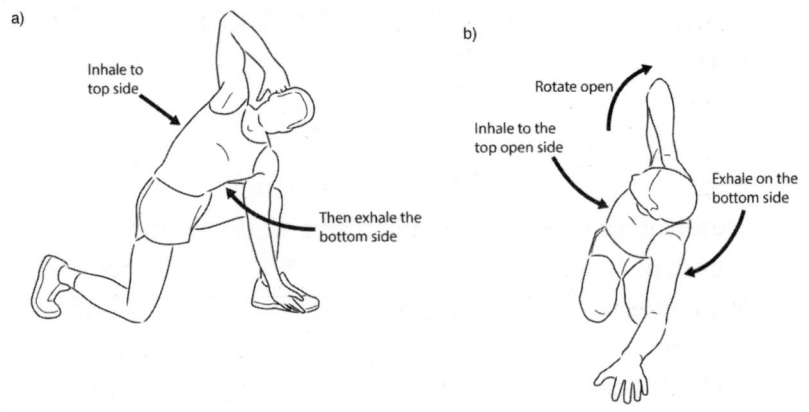

Your thoracic mobilisations can be done in something like a lunge, or in our test position

Just let it all hang out!

The impact of improving your breathing mechanics to help with hip tightness and reducing pain when running can happen faster than you might think, even immediately. One example of this was at a workshop for recreational runners that I taught in Scotland. At the end of the workshop, two middle-aged female runners came to me, a little bit shy and sheepish, to ask a question. There's some hesitancy as if they've just learned something about breathing that was total alien to them, or different from what they'd been doing their whole life. They asked: 'So, am I not supposed to be actively tensing my core when I'm running? Because when I run, I brace my core, and then I can't do the diaphragmatic breathing you just did with us.'

'Too much tension in your core reduces your ability for the lower ribs to move and therefore your diaphragm to function optimally. When you are overly tensing your abs, you are literally restricting your inhalation,' I replied, hoping they understood what the two-hour workshop was about, and I hadn't just wasted their time.

My mind flashed back to the conversations with physiotherapist Gemma Jefferson. *I bet their hips are tight*, I thought. If they are holding all that tension in the core and not using diaphragmatic breathing while running, those hips flexors and hips will tighten up to provide the stability.

I asked, 'Do you have tight hips?'

'Yes! Bane of our lives,' they both replied, almost excitedly as they started to understand there may be a link here with their breathing.

'Did they feel looser and release after we did the breathing mechanics exercise?' I asked.

'Oh yes, so much!' Sandra replied.

Bingo.

The tension in the core these two runners were creating was affecting their running form – a big mistake many runners make because core stability is often misunderstood and poorly taught. Restricting the lower ribs and overly tensing the core meant they had to breathe from the upper chest. That kept them in a vicious loop of poor breathing, tight hips and unable to relax when they ran.

'So we just have to let it all hang out. . . ?' Yep, let your breathing dynamics create the stability. It's more efficient, it's optimal for your movement and it's more economical than tensing your abs. It's almost like 'free' stability through air pressure (like in Gemma's canister), whereas tensing your abs takes, effort, energy, vital oxygen and restricts your diaphragm.

One week later I got an email from Sandra saying, 'I did the Baxter's 10km at the weekend with zero hip pain, I'm just delighted. So thankful I went to your workshop and discovered the benefits.'

Putting it into practice

Two areas to focus on from this chapter as we use these breathing techniques to become stronger runners are: First, use breathing mobilisations to free up your ribs, integrating them into your warm-ups. It can help free up your hips, spine and shoulders before you start warming up and it helps activate your breathing muscles. Second, experiment with how you link your breathing with your steps when running.

At the start I never was a fan of linking my breathing with any particular stride pattern or cadence. It felt restrictive to me. It felt like what James Earls explained was a benefit for humans being able to dissociate the movement of breathing from the movement of running. Linking them back up felt like a backward step in evolution. I tried it years ago, didn't like it, so simply shelved it as a 'not for me'. But if you feel the same initially, don't give up – it's worth sticking with it a little bit and giving it a chance. Initially just try it every now and again, before getting into the details of specific ratios in chapter 13. You don't always have to do it but I've found that in certain situations, such as easy runs or going up steep climbs, it gives me a focus, helps regulate pace, and I can relax more as I fall into flow state, and running just feels easier.

Two final points to be aware of with LRC. Firstly, by synchronising your breathing with your steps, you could be altering your cadence and stride length. For this reason, researchers advocate adjusting your breathing to match your step count, rather than altering your steps to match your breathing. Keep your stride length and cadence as you're used to, and instead play with your breath to find the ratio of breaths to step you enjoy.[15]

The final point is that trying out LRC in your next running session is not a trivial task. There is a certain additional cognitive challenge at the start due to the concentration and focus demands. The additional concentration might outweigh the physiological benefits, so it might not feel better at first. Hence the encouragement from me to not dismiss it straight away if it feels awkward or restrictive. Make a fair assessment of its use for you once you've had some practice and it feels more natural.

We noted at the start our diaphragm is more than just a breathing muscle – it can help transform your running by its effect on movement of the ribcage, spine and hips. Stability is one of its important functions. If you are not creating stability in your 'canister' through breathing diaphragmatically, then your body will find a way of creating that stability for you. Around your hips that means stiffening and tightening up your hip flexors, which you keep stretching with no success. It could 'switch off' your glutes, reduce your stride length and leave you with pain in the hips, knees, back or foot (or anywhere). Until we address breathing, we might always be restricted and swimming upstream.

The good news is now you have simple breathing mobilisation exercises, you can start using them straight away. The other thing is it doesn't get any more complicated. Breathing will start to be easier and easier, and your ribcage will start to expand more with less effort.

When we start to get more of the little things right, and not making mistakes like tensing our abs or repeatedly landing on the same leg at the end of an exhale, our aches and pains start to vanish, as the ladies from the Scotland workshop found, and countless other athletes I've worked with.

Key takeaways

- Your tight hip flexors won't release until you address your breathing dynamics and create stability in your 'canister', allowing you to relax your stomach and hip flexors.
- We can use our breath in warm-ups to mobilise the ribcage, helping free up the thoracic spine and hips.
- LRC links your breathing with your running cadence, which elites do naturally, providing free energy for your breathing muscles and a rhythm to hypnotise you into flow state.
- Odd numbers of foot strikes to breath cycles means your foot strikes swap on each exhale when you have the least pressure and stability in your system, which helps to reduce pain.

Seeing so much practical advice from Jacko on breathing has done so much for my running and general training. The daily habit of using it for nervous system regulation is building steadily. Thank you for everything you're putting into the world, it's mega!

Jack Manners, recreational runner

CHAPTER 10

More efficient with less oxygen

We're about to take our efficiency to new heights from two different angles. We're going to learn how fascia uses less oxygen and how our ribcage is essential for torquing up that fascia for more efficient running form. We'll also get some practise in getting accustomed to less oxygen that will take your breath away!

Don't try harder, use less oxygen

'Be as energy efficient as possible, use as little oxygen as necessary to save energy,' Shane Benzie encouraged me during our running session where he used video analysis to critique my technique. 'You run like a muscle man, Jacko.' Part of me likes Shane Benzie's description of my running. 'I'm skinny these days, mate, too much running! I'd have hated you to have seen me back when I played rugby!'

We both laughed at my poor attempt to glide in a relaxed fashion around the sports field where Shane is used to providing video analysis for much more aesthetically pleasing running form. I was keen to learn from Shane's wisdom and experience, as he's worked with some of the greatest runners in the world. Plus he has a unique take on observing and analysing movement.

He described to me that my self-perception of being muscular was stopping me relaxing. And when you're not relaxed, you can't be fluid, and when you're not being fluid, you miss out on the 'free energy' within the elasticity of your fascia. If you want to be more efficient with running, you need to use the fascia in the system, 'It's how the East Africans run, and it's why they are hard to catch!' Shane explained it simply, 'Muscles take up more oxygen to create force whereas the fascia is elastic and that elastic energy doesn't want oxygen like muscles do.'

Muscles don't just require more oxygen compared with the fascia; they also create lots of carbon dioxide and other by-products of cellular respiration. The body has to process and metabolise these by-products, which increases your urge to breathe and how much air you need to ventilate.

Shane explained, 'There are three key things runners get excited about: Lactate threshold, VO_2 max and running economy. They are less excited about economy until runners really understand it.' According to Shane, the East African runners he studied exploited this system, and, as a result, literally need less oxygen to run.

If I could improve the efficiency of my breathing and then combine that with the efficiency of my movement through improved running form, I'd be flying, I immediately thought. More fascia and less muscles mean less demand for oxygen, so it will be easier to stay calm and relaxed with my breathing, and therefore relaxed in body and mind – that was my theory. *Are there any links between what creates good posture for breathing and what's necessary for good running posture and form?*

Relaxation is still the key

Every running coach I'd spoken to had always emphasised the most important thing was to be relaxed. Shane shed new light on this, explaining why. Pointing at my six pack, he explained that tension, particularly in the stomach, affects posture and running form and, according to Shane, even my perception of myself will affect my running form. The tension around our core that Shane observes restricting posture and running form is the same tension performance physiotherapist Gemma described restricting our breathing – interesting!

The other thing that stops you from being relaxed is feeling out of breath. Shane explained that you can't move well if you're struggling for air. You need to be 'relaxed, fluid and rhythmic'. He noted that when learning new running techniques, the runner either holds their breath because of the cognitive challenge or their breathing becomes faster and shallower. Neither of which aid relaxation.

I briefly explained Gemma Jefferson's concept of the canister and the effect on the hip flexors to Shane and he agreed. He said, 'I get really excited about bio-tensegrity; everything is connected to everything, no dividing lines, only connecting lines. When you get the right posture and the right amount of tension into all those tendons and ligaments, that's going to create a more connected system that moves more easily.'

I was mesmerised by the way Shane sees and describes how he looks at the movement of a runner. 'I look at movement and explain it through anatomy, rather than using anatomy to try and explain movement. Our movement is based heavily on our perception of movement and that is heavily influenced by our understanding of biomechanics. Those that move most beautifully often don't know anything about anatomy and biomechanics. You look at an East African runner, they look like they're 7 foot tall and their legs come up to their neck. They run like the top of the leg isn't the top of the femur. That's because psoas major runs all the way up to T12. I think of the psoas muscle as the top of the leg, not where the femur goes into the hip, like our anatomy books.'

Shane saw the top of the leg as where psoas inserts to T12 at the bottom of the thoracic spine. Guess which muscle it intersects with there? Yep, the diaphragm. Does a well-functioning diaphragm help the function of psoas, allowing us to run with fluidity and seemingly longer legs? I was keen to understand what shape or posture Shane believed runners should get into to optimise running economy and the elasticity in the fascia.

He explained, 'Get in a beautiful position, height in the body through centre line from belly button to top of the head, opening a bow in that centre line, get hips forward and pelvis in a neutral position and load the elastic fascial system.' Based on Shane's biotensegrity model, if runners get into this shape, they create tension in the system that allows for efficient elastic movement and uses less oxygen.

The diaphragm is part of that fascial system. It is central to the deep front line, identified by Thomas Myers, author of *Anatomy Trains*. When we optimise the position of the ribcage, the diaphragm generates beneficial pressure in the canister. This pressure provides stability (allowing core and hip flexors to relax) and helps improve force transfer through the kinetic chain, reducing energy leaks within the fascial system when the foot strikes the ground. The good news is, as I discovered during our coaching session, the positioning of your ribcage for better breathing is the same position Shane described for better running.

Mistakenly, people often lean back and push the chest forward, which puts pressure on the lower back. This forward projected and tilted position of the ribcage also negatively affects ventilation and diaphragm function. From time spent with Shane, I realised that the shapes and posture he wants runners to get into for better running form and economy were the same shape and postures that I'm striving for with the ribcage to optimise breathing.

Shane concluded: 'I feel like we are saying the same thing but coming from two different angles.'

If you've done your homework from the last chapter with some of the breathing mobilisation drills at the start of your warm-ups, you might have noticed that breathing and expansion of your ribcage feels easier. Very simply, the stiffer your ribcage, the harder it is to expand and breathe, as well as achieve thoracic extension for that tall running posture. As we reduce stiffness and restore mobility to the ribcage, it's easier to get into that tall shape. Breathing is easier and good running form is easier. You use less oxygen when you're more efficient at both. It's another piece of the puzzle to becoming a stronger runner by breathing smarter.

Why hold your breath?

We've learned that being more efficient with running is about relying more on fascia than muscles so you don't need to use as much oxygen. What about getting used to not needing as much oxygen? What would that look like, is it something we can train?

Remember Emil Zátopek, the 'Czech locomotive', regarded as one of the greatest distance runners of all time? He won four Olympic gold medals and set 18 world records. He was the first runner ever to break the 29-minute mark in the 10,000m and in 1952 was the first, and only person ever, to win the 5000m, 10,000m and marathon at the same Olympics games, breaking the marathon record by six minutes in the process (which was even more impressive since it was the first time he'd run a marathon)!

He was well known for his brutal training sessions, which included holding his breath and running as far as he could to make it harder. Was he practising getting used to running with less oxygen by holding his breath?

Emil Zátopek isn't the only one. In his book *Hypoventilation Training*, French researcher Xavier Woorons writes that in the 1980s, the Brazilian coach Luiz De Oliveria used breath-holding with his athletes once a week, notably 800m Olympic champion Joaquim Cruz and 1500 and 3000m World Champion Marie Decker.[1]

Xavier Woorons is a pioneer in hypoventilation (reduced breathing) training, where he uses breath-holding with athletes to elicit an additional training response.

It sounds like an oxymoron because when you hold your breath, you are starving your body of oxygen; your ventilation drops to zero because you're not breathing. How on earth can that be helpful, is a sensible question to ask!

In the short term – while holding your breath – it is not a performance enhancer; it may even limit your performance depending on the type of running session. But it's the adaptations it creates in the long term. It's a tool you can use in a training session to see benefits later.

During breath-holding, one of the stimuli we're looking to create is a drop in oxygen within the bloodstream (blood oxygen saturation) and therefore less available oxygen reaches the working muscles (muscle oxygenation) – essentially, you are practising needing less oxygen.

Its technical name in sports science is hypoxic (low oxygen) training, and has been well researched for the past couple of decades. I'd totally forgotten about my first experience of hypoxic training. Partly because it was part of a charity Red Nose Day event and partly because it was over 15 years ago, but mainly because I had no experience or even interest in hypoxic training. It was held at England Football's training facility, St George's Park, where they had a conditioning chamber that altered the amount of available oxygen as a percentage in the chamber. Normal atmosphere percentage of oxygen is 20.9%, whereas for this charity event, they had me and a former professional footballer on a Wattbike at the equivalent of the top of Mount Everest. Needless to say, after only a few seconds of pedalling on the Wattbike, I was completely out of breath, gasping for air that didn't feel like it was there. It was alarming how out of breath I was considering how much cycling I was doing. My perception of effort was disjointed, and it made me panic. We all had a bit of a laugh about it afterwards. I can't even remember the purpose of the challenge. I thought no more about it until reading Xavier Woorons's work explaining you can create a hypoxic training environment not with fancy expensive chambers but by simply holding your breath.

Training adaptations

Interestingly, the ability to hold your breath and exercise, as well as deal with the physiological and psychological discomfort, is a trainable process. Individuals who practise breath-holding get better at breath-holding. Not only do they get better at dealing with the psychological discomfort by pushing mental boundaries, physiologically, their body becomes accustomed to the lack of oxygen and learns to adapt. The body's response to hypoxia is trainable. You get better at holding your breath, and the body gets better at responding.

The short-term response from the body to a longer breath-hold that creates a greater drop in oxygen is the contraction of the spleen.

The spleen is like a blood bank, storing around 8% more red blood cells, which are rich in haemoglobin, helping to improve oxygen transport and circulation of oxygen upon release. It's a temporary fix for the body rather than a long-term adaptation, as the spleen reabsorbs those red blood cells. It makes sense: the spleen contracts in response to hypoxia. What's cool is that training affects the extent to which the spleen contracts. Individuals trained in breath-holding have a stronger response and contraction of the spleen than untrained individuals.

What is the point of this? Does it help you run better, faster or further? Well, having more haemoglobin-rich red blood cells circulating in your bloodstream increases the oxygen-carrying capacity of the blood, improving the oxygen transport that we typically think of as automatic and untrainable (without doping – naughty). The most recent study on this as I write is from 2024, where experienced runners performed five maximal breaths before a graded exercise test to exhaustion on a treadmill and compared it with a baseline test, without the five breath-holds as a warm-up.[2] The results showed 'significant increases in haematocrit, haemoglobin concentration, red blood cell count, and muscle deoxygenation, accompanied by a reduction in blood lactate concentration.' They retested to exhaustion with all that additional haematocrit, haemoglobin, red blood cells and less lactate in the system. The researchers observed 'a significantly delayed onset time of the second ventilatory threshold and increased time to exhaustion.' Pretty impressive for a short-term breath-holding intervention!

Before you get excited and start trying to hold your breath before running sessions, there are more benefits that I want to explain because they are longer-term adaptations for your red blood cells, rather than just a short-term hack.

Longer-term adaptations

One of the observations Xavier Woorons noted is that the main long-term benefits from training breath-holds during exercise are improved performance and faster recovery, in anaerobic rather than aerobic training. This is because the main benefits are improving lactate tolerance and reoxygenation in recovery periods from interval training or repeated hill runs or sprints.

He has carried out extensive research into the adaptations following exhale breath-holds combined with repeated-sprint training. His 2018 study saw an astonishing 10-fold improvement over a four-week trial of training repeated sprints over 40m.[3]

In the study they established a baseline of how many 40m sprints the subjects could complete every 30 seconds (each sprint lasting around six seconds, with 24 seconds of rest between sprints). The test ended once their velocity dropped below 85% of their maximum, and the total number of 40m sprints recorded.

The group that completed four weeks of breath-holding training on an exhale during their sprint training (twice per week) improved from 9.1 repetitions (average number of 40m sprints achieved) at the start to a staggering 14.9. A massive 64% improvement in the number of repeat sprints they could complete. Compared with only a 6% improvement, from 9.8 to 10.4 repetitions for the control group. That's 10 times the improvement over four weeks by simply holding their breath after an exhale. That's a crazy improvement in such a short training period.

How is that possible? What is the breath-hold doing to make so much improvement? I tracked Xavier Woorons down for an interview and he described the breath-holds as voluntary hypoventilation at low lung volume (VHL), meaning the breath-hold is performed at the end of an exhale. He believes there are two mechanisms responsible for the improvements after high-intensity or repeated-sprint training with voluntary hypoventilation at VHL:

1. 'A greater energy supply from the lactic anaerobic metabolism during sprints combined with greater lactate tolerance.'
2. 'A greater muscle reoxygenation during the recovery periods enabling higher elimination of waste metabolites, in particular the hydrogen ions produced by the higher glycolysis activity. Greater muscle reoxygenation also means greater lactate clearance, even though a high level of lactate concentration

is not considered a limiting factor during exercise, unlike the hydrogen ions which provoke blood and muscle acidosis.'

So, by training repeated sprints while holding your breath after an exhale, you can improve the anaerobic system and how your body tolerates and utilises lactate for energy. The breath-hold deprives the body of more oxygen than it's used to during sprints, meaning it relies on the anaerobic system to a greater degree, which increases the amount of lactate produced, hence the body adapts to improve how it uses and tolerates lactate. Greater lactate tolerance and utilisation during running can be very advantageous, resulting in improved ventilatory thresholds and reduced time to fatigue.

What about the improved recovery he's observed in his studies? Does starving the body of oxygen during the sprint by holding the breath actually help get more oxygen into the muscles afterwards? Xavier Woorons explains: 'Two mechanisms are likely to improve the oxygen supply to the muscles during the recovery periods of a repeated-sprint exercise after a high-intensity VHL training:'

1. 'An improved oxygen transport in the blood through higher cardiac output. In previous studies, we had indices that tend to show that stroke volume, which is an important factor of cardiac output, could be increased after VHL training. However, this has to be confirmed in further studies.'
2. 'A greater amount of blood, and therefore of oxygen, available for the muscles. On the other hand, so far, we have failed to find any improvement in oxygen extraction or utilization by the muscles after a VHL training. This result surprised us and contradicted our hypothesis. Therefore, this kind of method may induce more anaerobic than aerobic physiological adaptations at the muscle level.'

To summarise, more blood can be pumped from the heart, which helps to improve the delivery of oxygen to the muscles during the recovery periods. Also, improved reoxygenation during the recovery periods after training with exhale breath-holds helps with clearing waste metabolites, especially hydrogen ions, which increase acidity, leading to fatigue. It's almost as if the body gets better at driving oxygen back to the muscle as an adaptation when it's been exposed to some training with less available oxygen. At the same time, it improves its ability to deal with and process the waste products that normally lead to fatigue.

In Woorons's 2024 study, he attributed these results to 'enhanced muscle profusion' and 'a blood volume redistribution within the body'.[4] He noted that after a period of training exhale breath-holds with repeated sprints, 'it is likely that perfusion of other body territories, in particular the skin, were also reduced to cope with the increased amount of blood to the muscles'. The body is clever, right? It notices the increased hypoxia (low oxygen) in the working leg muscles from the exhale breath-hold sprints and diverts blood from less essential areas, such as the skin, to increase blood flow to the muscle lacking oxygen.

However, oxygen extraction did not appear to improve, contrary to expectations. If oxygen extraction improved at the muscle level, it would be advantageous for aerobic adaptations, whereas results indicate it is more beneficial for anaerobic training – such as repeated-sprint training, hill sprints and interval training potentially. Chapter 13 covers where best to use this type of training.

In addition to physiological adaptations from running with less oxygen, we also get used to controlling our urge to breathe when the breath-hold ends. The skill of controlling our breathing when we feel out of breath is a combination of physiological and psychological factors that we can train and improve. Controlling the urge to quickly expel the built-up carbon dioxide and gasp for fresh air following a breath-hold is one aspect. Others include the stress response induced by breath-holding, as it dampens vagal tone and increases sympathetic activation – it's up-regulating your ANS![5]

If we can get used to running with less oxygen, better control our urge to breathe and combine that with running more efficiently with posture that facilitates better ribcage position for more efficient breathing, we're starting to stack everything in our favour. The pieces of our breathing puzzle are taking shape.

Let's look at practical ways you can start improving your ribcage position for more efficient running and breath-holding.

Exercise: 'Chest up and ribs back'

The kingpin to good running form from Shane Benzie's wisdom is about getting the chest up, the spine tall and leading with sternum to create what he describes as a 'bow' to torque up and tense the fascia line from your head to your toe. No mention of the ribcage, but what is your chest? Where is your sternum? Your ribs connect into your sternum; it's part of the ribcage. We've already explained the relationship with the ribs and the spine in the last two chapters. When Shane says 'chest, spine and sternum', I think ribcage.

Getting your ribcage in the right position helps with efficient breathing and, at the same time, ticks off all the good running-form boxes. A tall position so the ribcage has freedom to expand and the diaphragm has space to move down towards the pelvis.

I simplify it down to these two cues: 'chest up, ribs back'.

It couldn't be any simpler, but it couldn't have a bigger impact on your breathing, your running and the relationship between the two. When the chest is up, the ribcage is open, the spine is long. When the ribs are back, the ribcage is stacked on top of the pelvis in good alignment, rather than projected forward, which is a common mistake.

If someone has flared ribs or projected ribcage because they lack thoracic extension, and the posterior ribs are all tight, restricted and jacked up, they will find it harder to create Shane's 'bow'. Even if they do get close to it, restrictions in the posterior ribs and resulting thoracic spine position means breathing mechanics are limited. They will likely overarch the back and roll the pelvis forwards, losing alignment between the ribcage and pelvis and reducing length through the spine. Hence the importance of the breathing mobilisations from the last chapter.

My best advice is to start using the two simple cues: 'chest up' and 'ribs back' when you are doing your warm-ups or easy runs. When you are not being challenged by the intensity of your running, it's a great chance to place some focus on your breathing. The simplest and best thing you can do for both your running posture and breathing is work on the position of your ribcage. Be aware, though, it might be a bit trickier than you think. Simple as it seems, Shane Benzie points out, 'breathing patterns love the rhythm of the body so they settle into the rhythm of the body. When moving differently the breathing patterns often change and alter. For example, when someone increases cadence, their breathing rate also increases to match the cadence increase.' So, we need to be careful with our breathing when trying to change, alter or improve running technique.

He continues, 'learning a new skill like altering running form is almost a perfect storm for being cardio-vascularly challenged; increased perception of effort, cognitively challenged and requiring more oxygen, asked to be more elastic but the fascia system isn't adapted yet, so they use more muscular effort which requires more oxygen.' It seems that not only is breathing important for everything we've already uncovered, it's also going to be challenged when we try to improve running form. We therefore need to have a good handle on our breathing and use it to help stay relaxed while working on technique, rather than panicking, feeling out of breath or even holding our breath when trying to improve our form.

Exercise: Exhale breath-holds

One exceptionally important thing to point out right at the start with any form of breath-holding is the safety component. Breath-holding creates a strong anaerobic stimulus to your training and is considered a stressor. Your heart rate will increase – we've seen from the research that it increases cardiac output – so it's important that you are fit and healthy, with no heart conditions, blood pressure issues (high or low), and don't suffer from panic attacks before using breath-holds in any training sessions.

It is key that breath-holds are done after an exhalation rather than an inhalation. If you hold your breath on an inhale after filling up the lungs, they're relatively rich in oxygen compared with holding on an exhale when the lungs are relatively empty of oxygen. Remember, we are trying to help the body adapt to working with less oxygen.

If you hold on an inhale, you'll be able to hold for longer. When oxygen is transferred into the working muscle tissues, the blood is replenished with oxygen from the lungs if they are full. Essentially, we are delaying the time before you start to have a meaningful reduction in oxygen supply. This is in contrast to holding the breath on the exhale (relatively empty lungs); when the oxygen that leaves the blood into the muscle tissues is not replenished from the lungs, you'll get to a lack of oxygen supply quicker and potentially a stronger hypoxic effect.

The final important factor Xavier Woorons points out from his research is that the breath-hold is 'maintained up to the breaking point'. Meaning the strong desire to breathe needs to be achieved to elicit the response and subsequent adaptations from the body. Or another way, to put it simply, if you don't try very hard and don't hold your breath for very long, then you won't create much of a training adaptation.

So how long is realistic to hold your breath while running?

Xavier Woorons suggested around seven to eight seconds is the maximum. However, factors such as the individual themselves, experience, running pace and terrain, as well as rest periods, all have an effect. I've personally seen elite athletes' improvements over time with training to exceed more than 10 seconds for repeated breath-hold sprints, suggesting it's a trainable process. Xavier Woorons explained in his research they never measured whether breath-hold time improves but he believes it is trainable, which he attributes to increased tolerance to hypercapnia (high carbon dioxide levels) and would help create stronger adaptations.

This highlights an important point of breath-hold training. Not only are we getting the body used to being comfortable with less oxygen, the greater tolerance to carbon dioxide can help with breath control when running. This is especially important at higher-intensity sessions or when we are really pushing our limits chasing PBs or Strava segments!

Starting with exhaling, holding your breath and running for six to eight seconds with a one-minute recovery between is a progressive way to get used to the sensation of breath-holding and running. It also gives you some practice in breath control: when the breath-hold ends, don't just let the air rush out and your chest pump up and down. Instead practise the skill of breathing better mechanically and controlling the speed of your breathing while you're feeling more out of breath than usual.

A couple of tips:

- Don't be surprised when you feel out of breath at the end of the breath-hold, you know it's coming, so when you finish the hold, be ready to act calm (think poker face) and use your good diaphragmatic breathing mechanics to help control the stronger urge to breathe.
- During the breath-hold itself, try to relax and try to swallow. The swallowing reflex is linked to your breathing and tricks your brain that everything is ok while you hold your breath and run!

They are great to do in warm-ups before your runs, and in chapter 13 we'll detail how to integrate them progressively into higher-intensity sessions to help turn you into your own 'locomotive beast' like Emil Zátopek.

Putting it into practice

The day after my running analysis session with Shane, I travelled down to teach a breath-training workshop in London. While driving, I couldn't stop thinking of simple but very profound tips Shane gave me from the video analysis of my running. I was trying to take my personal bias out of the thought process, as I believe breathing to be so important for running performance, efficiency and posture. But I couldn't get away from the fact that nearly everything he said about body position that was good for running technique, I would describe as good for breathing. If we improve breathing, we naturally get into better running postures – they seem to be connected. I was keen to try and combine the two to see how it affected my running: n =1 but 1 is infinitely better than zero.

I stopped at a small park near Oxford on the way, eager to just get out and start linking the new running technique tips from Shane with my breathing. I whipped off my trousers in the back of the campervan, slipped on my offensively short running shorts, put my running trainers on, and I was off.

By now, usually when I'm running, my focus would be on my breathing. Being aware of my diaphragm, sensing my ribcage expanding and keeping my airway nice and open with good tongue and neck positioning. But as I started running, I wasn't thinking about my breathing, I was laser-focused on my running technique. *Chest up, create that bow and push the ground away*, I kept saying to myself. *Oh, and relax*, that was the most important thing. But as soon as I thought about relaxation, I realised that I wasn't relaxed, I was too focused on trying to do the technique right. It felt a bit different.

I switched focus to my breathing: *how am I breathing? I'm nasal breathing and my ribcage feels nice and open with that chest position, but the air hunger is pretty strong, I feel a bit out of breath.* I was a bit confused, *I thought it was supposed to make this easier?* I checked the pace I was running at and was surprised to see a 4:15min/km pace. I was only just warming into the run and thought I was maybe running around a 6min/km pace. It gave me some confidence that I was on the right track. If I was running that fast (for me) but didn't realise or feel like I was trying hard, that's a good sign of efficiency. Maybe I was being more elastic and therefore running faster with less perceived or even actual effort. *I need to get better at relaxing into this new sensation of combining the running technique and breathing technique.* I thought about what coaches Shane Benzie and Dr Martin Yelling said about relaxation being the most important thing.

I was reminded of the interview with the world champion freediver, Davide Carrera, explaining that to calm our breathing response we have to calm the mind. Too much thinking takes up too much vital oxygen for a freediver to hold their breath underwater and swim to a depth of 100m and back up on a single breath. Thinking takes energy. Thinking uses oxygen. And I was thinking too much. After a short break I set off with an intention to not think but to let the technique tips 'just happen', not overanalyse it or my breathing. Simply relax into any sensations my breath created and let my body be fluid.

I completed a few more laps and at some point, towards the end I felt like I was flying along. My pace was 3:40min/km! Wow, for me that is fast. The session was a bit stop–start, as I was playing with the technique, but I covered around 5km in total. I got back to the campervan with a smile on my face because I remember a time just three years ago when I was running around Gedling country park while preparing for my first marathon. At that point I was focused purely on my breathing. To be able to feel in control of my breathing and maintain nasal breathing without feeling stressed by the air hunger, I had to run at a 6:30min/km pace. That's not particularly fast is it? It's more like jogging. Gradually, with adaptation, I'd increased my comfortable pace to 5:30min/km pace, and when training for the Eryri Marathon, I was hitting 5min/km for some 10km training runs and a half marathon. But just now, without time for adaptation, just linking running technique and breathing technique, I was at 3:40min/km. I actually felt like a runner. Not only had my running changed, my perception of self had changed too.

Becoming more efficient

If you want to try and become a more efficient runner, a more efficient breather who needs less oxygen, one of the best tools is breath-holding after an exhalation while running. Xavier Woorons recommends only two breath-hold training sessions a week and it is most important to consider the following: 'VHL training is a demanding method, the VHL sessions should not be preceded or followed within the 24 hours by high-intensity training (with normal breathing). While VHL training can be beneficial for improving performance when all parameters are managed correctly, it can also be counterproductive when this is not the case.'

Therefore, we need to respect the intensity of adding exhale breath-hold training sessions into our weekly running schedule and plan them around other high-intensity or threshold-style sessions. The recovery protocols in chapter 12 will also come in handy to help offset the extra stress the breath-hold sessions might add to your training load. Remember you get better when you adapt, and that means you have to recover. But don't worry, as well as adding intensity to your training sessions like this, we also have the tools to help you improve your recovery.

There's an opportunity to start combining everything we've been learning about thus far. Get your ribcage mobilised in warm-ups, get the chest up and ribs back when running, and try some breath-holds in your warm-ups to start with. As you begin adding all these little pieces of the puzzle together, you use more tools, get better at using them and gradually adapt to be a stronger, more efficient runner.

We've learned how our ribcage can be the kingpin to more efficient running form and it's the same ribcage position we want for efficient breathing. A more efficient running posture that utilises the fascia instead of muscles uses less vital oxygen. If we are breathing more efficiently too, then we don't need as much air or need to breathe as fast to oxygenate sufficiently. This means breathing requires less effort, which helps with that all-important sense of relaxation.

Key takeaways

- Breathing and running form are linked by the good posture required to optimise them, and the ribcage is central to both.
- When you are efficient at breathing and running, you use less oxygen at a relative pace.
- Breath-holding in training can create strong physiological and psychological adaptations.
- Research has shown that breath-holding is a simple technique to help improve lactate utilisation, tolerance and clearance and enhance muscle reoxygenation in recovery periods.

Breath training has opened up another dimension to the work we do with our footballers. It's enhanced multiple areas such as our mobility, CV and recovery work. Through working with Jacko we've been able to meet the needs of the team with greater breadth and depth, resulting in performance enhancement and greater well-being. It's a discipline that when taught, understood and engaged with well can bring real positive change and growth for our footballers in many areas of their health and performance.

Fran Clarkson, lead physiotherapist, England Women's Football

CHAPTER 11

When the nose isn't enough

There's a time for everything. There's a time and a place for nasal breathing during running, but there are also times when your nose may not allow you to oxygenate sufficiently. When you are really pushing the running pace, you may need to use the bigger hole in your face, but not as a compensation. We're about to optimise your mouth breathing, which includes a game-changing hack!

Have we changed the auto setting?

On a cold but crisp afternoon in Eryri National Park (Snowdonia), I had a run in mind where I wanted to test my new breathing philosophy. It was 11 November 2024 and I had Moel Tryfan in my sights. He's the little brother of the daunting 917m-tall Tryfan, which sits in the main mountain range. Moel Tryfan stands at just 427m. With a 5km loop from my front door, it posed a short but challenging climb. There are a number of routes up, but on that day, I had the taste for a route that takes you straight up the steepest ascent. On Strava the segment is appropriately named 'Moel Tryfan direct'.

    I wanted to see how I'd fare if I didn't try and force any particular breathing pattern or control and relied on the training habits and adaptations I'd made over the last couple of months. By now my diaphragm was strong, and it functioned naturally even when mouth breathing during running (I'd earned the right to mouth breathe). I'd been working hard on my carbon dioxide tolerance with plenty of NT and exhale breath-hold training, as well as changing my perception of self, effort and air hunger.

I took it steady on the first couple of kilometres, relaxing into nasal breathing as I came up the gradual incline, past the old slag heaps of seemingly unlimited piles of the famous purple Snowdonia slate, to the approach of the daunting Moel Tryfan direct. I maintained nasal breathing in the first part of the approach, but the incline turns aggressively steep almost immediately, and the drowning sensation from the air hunger was about to smack me in the face. I trusted my process: *Let's see what all this training has created, then.*

The mouth opened, and I just put my head down and kept driving my feet into the floor. It's the type of incline in the mountains that when I previously attempted it, I had to stop three or four times. A year ago, there was no way I could run up this without stopping to walk for some part of it. Breathing was hard and heavy. My heart rate peaked at 177bpm (my max is 183bpm from my VO_2 max test). It was hard but surprisingly manageable. I was excited but probably more relieved. I really wanted all of the breath training to have paid off. I wanted to show myself that I'd changed my auto and not only did it feel relatively 'hard but okay' – probably the type of 'how it's supposed to feel' that Math Roberts spoke of – I got to the top without stopping to walk. I didn't manage top spot on the Strava segment – it belongs to a certain Math Roberts (I couldn't believe it, but I did get second place). It was like when Roger Black felt like he'd won when he got silver at the 1996 Olympic games because it was unrealistic to beat the infamous Michael Johnson! In fact, I'd gone much quicker, completing the short segment in just 3:29 rather than my previous attempt of 4:29, a whole minute faster, and I actually felt better when I got to the top, more in control, more relaxed – I'd just run up a mountain!

My philosophy of 'earn the right to mouth breathe' rather than it being a compensation had worked. It made sense. I was going faster and at a more intense pace on a demanding incline than I could manage with my nose, but through adaptation, I was able to benefit from the efficiency we've learned that nasal breathing provides, but using my mouth. Opening up what felt like a sixth gear, when I'd been used to a car with only five.

Just because we open the mouth, doesn't mean we open the floodgates to fast, shallow, inefficient breathing

It's safe to say the vast majority of us won't be able to do all of our running with nasal breathing, especially during high-intensity and paced runs. The research we've seen suggests that with training most people can achieve up to 80% or even 85% of our VO_2 max breathing nasally, which can be as high as over 90% of our maximum heart rate. But what about when you are working harder, at a higher intensity? Forcing nasal breathing beyond your current nasal threshold can limit your performance. The ventilation you require at that point might be greater than you can manage with your nose, potentially leading to inadequate oxygenation if you are truly under-breathing (hypoventilating). At that point, forcing nasal breathing isn't just not relaxing, it can feel like you are suffocating or drowning – I've been there! You could actually be limiting the vital oxygen getting to your muscles, as well as the clearance of waste metabolites.

From the assessments in chapter 7, hopefully you have an idea of your switching point from nasal to mouth breathing. Remember, your NT will change based on things outside of your control, like weather conditions or inclines and even stress levels or the menstrual cycle. It will also improve and increase in time as you increase your carbon dioxide tolerance, reduce your perception of air hunger, and increase the strength and capacity of your diaphragm and associated breathing muscles.

Opening your mouth at that point is not just what you might do intuitively, but it is also necessary. But when it opens, what you do with it and how you manage the speed of your breathing and the function of your diaphragm are two vital factors that directly impact the efficiency of your mouth breathing, which you need to be aware of. In time and after putting in the work to 'earn the right to mouth breathe', you'll naturally benefit from the diaphragm drawing air into the lower portion of the lungs. This is a naturally slower process than relying on shallow upper chest panting, which usually happens when you're forced to mouth breathe, if you lack understanding and practice of optimal breathing patterns.

What to do when you switch to the mouth

When you choose to switch to the mouth is up to you, but don't force it. You have a couple of hacks, such as turtle power or Vassos Alexander's 'power of the smile', to help the nostrils stay open. They can help increase ventilation with your nose by potentially 26%. If you force nasal breathing, you'll lose relaxation and can even increase heart rate and cardiovascular stress, turning running into a stressful experience. Hence, 'preference of the participant should be the determining factor . . . during competition and higher-intensity exercise' according to a 2017 study.[1]

There are three key things to keep in mind to maintain good breathing efficiency when you switch to mouth breathing, which will help prevent you from slipping into old compensatory habits:

- Always use your diaphragm.
- Make the mouth work like a nose.
- Exhales are where the magic is.

Always use your diaphragm (that's its job)

The most important of those is the use of your diaphragm. Potentially more important than which hole in your face you use. Your diaphragm is like the key domino that knocks over most of the rest. When you use your diaphragm, it takes longer, which means a slower, more controlled breathing rate (relatively) and a deeper breath due to the location of the diaphragm at the bottom of the ribcage. Your mechanics are better when you are using your diaphragm and it's likely so too is your control of breathing rate. You get to benefit from improved alveoli ventilation and ventilation efficiency by harnessing this in training.

Make the mouth work like a nose

There are a couple of things to be aware of when you switch to mouth breathing. One is that your mouth provides less resistance than your nose, so it's much easier for the upper chest and associated secondary breathing muscles to hike the ribcage up to take over. The other thing is that the brain likes tasks that are easy and familiar. Without awareness, education or understanding, it's likely any previous mouth breathing you've done while running will have been linked to a dominant upper chest breathing pattern with less recruitment of the diaphragm. The brain will take the path of least resistance, so it's the likely auto you'll slip into if you are not aware. Just because it's automatic doesn't mean it's optimal, remember.

We've also mentioned previously that this type of breathing pattern is your body's way to get you to stop and preserve itself (Central Governor Theory). Neurologically, it's also what your brain is used to when you breathe through the mouth, so, you have habits associated with that. Habits creating neural firing pathways as well as patterns developed within your fascia and muscles. It can feel like you're fighting a losing battle when you try to alter it at the start.

We can, however, use our newfound understanding to appreciate that the resistance of the nose is what helps towards recruitment of the diaphragm – not only that, tongue position is also key. You can't have your tongue up in the palate while mouth breathing because it blocks the mouth airway. Hence one of my favourite coaching cues for when we switch to mouth breathing is: 'make your mouth work like a nose'!

This means make your mouth smaller; don't have it wide open as you further reduce the resistance and you're more likely to drop into fast panting and lose control of your breathing rate. When your breathing rate spirals out of control, you lose tidal volume, your heart rate increases and you are in a vicious cycle of fast, shallow panting until you stop running.

Look at someone like Eliud Kipchoge. When he comes in to break an 'impossible' two-hour marathon, his mouth is open, he's smiling. But is it hanging wide open and panting? No! His mouth is open a small amount; he's certainly not out of breath and even looks like he could have done a sprint finish. It's even difficult to say whether he's exclusively breathing through his mouth or nose. Sometimes his mouth is shut, sometimes open a little, sometimes he might be using a bit of mouth and nose combined. But it's always relaxed and his run looks almost effortless.

So, make your mouth work like a nose. Have it open a smaller amount and allow it to provide a little bit of resistance. Enough that you can feel your diaphragm engaged, but not so much you can't relax. You are in control of how wide you open your mouth. Start with a smaller opening and gradually increase if you need to. Give it some time and you'll change your auto, and you won't need to think about it, it will just happen. How long will that take? I can't say. But what I can say, is that it feels amazing when you are cruising along at a faster pace than you've ever maintained before, and you can simply relax knowing that you're breathing efficiently, despite having to open your mouth. You feel in control and your diaphragm working. It's a magical feeling. You're relaxed.

As well as having the option to gradually open your mouth wider and wider if needed at higher intensities, you also have the option to use your nose and mouth together. Some people have adopted this approach and called it 'breathing gears'. Many people use this description and protocol that was first developed by Brian MacKenzie, an endurance athlete, coach and author. The lowest gear being nose inhale and nose exhale, increasing to nose inhale, mouth exhale, before reaching mouth inhale and mouth exhale. For some runners it can feel a bit too prescriptive and therefore restrictive, but there are intricacies between and within these gears that you can utilise so they become more 'flexible' rather than 'set' gears. How active the inhale and exhales are, for example, or how long the inhale or exhales last. What I'd like to bring to your attention is the critical point that whatever strategy you take, remaining in control of your breathing rate and engaging your diaphragm is the most important thing.

The main gear to highlight in this chapter is the middle gear (nasal inhale, mouth exhale). When you feel like you have to open your mouth because the air hunger is becoming too much and you can't relax. You can make an informed decision that you'll maintain nasal inhales but use your mouth for the exhale, which will allow for a greater volume of carbon dioxide to be expelled faster. As more carbon dioxide is removed faster than you can comfortably manage nasally, you might find that this strategy is enough to allow you to stay relaxed and reduce the sensation of air hunger. In that scenario you get the best of both worlds. With the inhale, you benefit from the nose, but you don't feel restricted by the carbon dioxide build-up as you let it out of the mouth on the exhale.

Exhales are where the magic is

It might appear a little ironic that in this section the emphasis is on the exhalation over the inhalation. We often think and focus on the inhale when our breathing feels uncomfortable and we're out of breath on a run. Yet the magic is in the exhale because that's where the carbon dioxide is.

We've already touched on the fact that one of the key drivers behind the perception of air hunger and feeling out of breath is rising carbon dioxide levels. You can't get rid of it fast enough when the levels exceed your tolerance, which leads to faster breathing rates, and we usually lose relaxation. In the long term, we want to dampen the response of those chemoreceptors to carbon dioxide with tolerance training. However, that takes time, but there are a few tricks we can keep up our sleeve.

This isn't a new concept. In 1986 Ian Jackson (no relation to me, so no bias!) published a book called *The Breathplay Approach to Whole Life Fitness*, where the emphasis of his breathing technique was on the exhalation rather than the inhalation.[2]

A 1987 study tested the effect of Jackson's Breathplay technique on trained cyclists.[3] They found that the 'forceful expiration and less forceful inspirations in varying ratios' produced some wild performance benefits. One group of cyclists completed three days of training with 12 hours of coaching to learn the technique. 'Significant gains' were recorded in time to exhaustion, versus control (7.2% improvement v 0%), decrease in submaximal heart rate (4.7% v 2.8%) and RPE (9.6% v 4.6%). Anaerobic threshold was delayed by two minutes but unchanged for the control group.

Most notable was the effect on carbon dioxide. In the Breathplay group, peak carbon dioxide levels were reached 26.8% later versus 14.8% earlier for the control group. Submaximal volume of carbon dioxide decreased by 9.8% versus 0.8%. The forceful exhalations were helping to delay the critical point where carbon dioxide becomes a problem for our breathing, heart rate and feeling of exhaustion. The researchers concluded that this technique helps 'increase endurance and delay onset of anaerobic threshold'.[4] More recently, researchers have looked back at Ian Jackson's technique, and although more research is needed, they suggest that the positive pressures created during the forced exhales may also help improve cardiac output during more intense running, thus sending more blood and oxygen to your muscles.[5]

Breathing efficiently with the mouth

Hopefully that's enough encouragement about the importance of exhales and the magic they have hidden within them for you to take exhales seriously. What does it look like in practical terms and how can you use it to your advantage?

The next steps can transform your higher-intensity running as we combine a few principles. Firstly, we need to be able to exhale well to do it forcefully. It's worth pointing out at this stage it could, of course, be done through the nose, but it tends to be less effective in practice. The time to apply this strategy is when the nose isn't enough and you are working at a greater intensity than your NT. Using the mouth for the forceful exhales is where the magic is at, as you'll clear more carbon dioxide efficiently via the larger hole in your face.

That said, for it to be forceful we need a few more pieces of our puzzle in place. We need to make the mouth smaller to create some level of resistance that encourages engagement of the exhalation muscles, especially the internal and external obliques. Your ability to engage those active exhalation muscles comes down to two things; how strong are those muscles, and how tight are the ribs in order to move 'downwards and inwards' (internal rotation and flexion) to expel the air. If your ribcage is restricted, the intercostal muscles between the ribs are tight and the muscles that move them are weak, so forceful exhalation will be tough – you'll compensate with spinal flexion that will upset your tall running form. You'll feel weak on exhalation and it won't be effective. You'll say it doesn't work; you'll dismiss the results from the study as 'a small sample size' and you'll miss out on the magic in your exhales.

Therefore, it's very important to have mobilised your ribs to be able to engage your active exhalation muscles without compensation, as shown in the 'exhale floor bridge' exercise in chapter 9. Once you can exhale well without compensating, you can start to try integrating it into running sessions when you feel like you're becoming a bit out of breath.

It's a good idea to practise it before you start feeling out of breath on a run because by the time the air hunger is strong, it's much harder to regain control of your breathing – but I do have a hack for you at the end of this chapter too. Don't worry, I've always got your back!

Once settled into your running, it's very helpful to use the forced exhales to find a rhythm. This is most effectively done by syncing those active exhales with your steps, as LRC outlined in chapter 9. By syncing the forced exhales with your steps, you benefit from both balancing carbon dioxide levels and delaying fatigue, as described in the Breathplay technique, as well as from the improved relaxation and 'rebound' of the inhale reported with LRC.

Timing those exhales with your foot strike once you're in a rhythm – and the number of strides per exhale that suits your carbon dioxide tolerance – helps you fall into relaxation and you won't feel out of breath. You know you're working hard, but you don't feel the same level of fatigue because you don't feel out of breath. It's almost surprising at first, and it feels a bit strange in a way to be working hard but not feeling out of breath. But strange in a good way, magical almost.

The hack: The CO_2 dump

They say, 'save the best for last', which might be the case when you feel the effect of a CO_2 dump or two! It does exactly what it says on the tin. It's a dump of carbon dioxide. The purpose of it is to offload excessive carbon dioxide that's built up because your running intensity is beyond your current carbon dioxide tolerance threshold to the point where you can't control your breathing. When you feel completely out of breath you spiral into the worst pattern of fast, mouth breathing and shallow panting. That's when it's appropriate to get rid of the gas that's causing the issue. Dump off the excess carbon dioxide.

It's important to dump as efficiently and effectively as possible to return to good breathing patterns to oxygenate your depleted muscles quickly. So again, we use the mouth as it allows us to offload a larger volume of carbon dioxide in each dump. We do it as quickly and explosively as possible. Again, you'll need those good active exhales you developed from the exhale floor bridge drill.

> **TRY THIS**
>
> When dumping carbon dioxide:
> - Don't worry about the inhale, let that just rebound naturally.
> - Use the mouth to force as much air out as quickly as possible; don't slow or extend the exhale at all.
> - Let the inhale rebound but get back to the next carbon dioxide dump as quickly as feels naturally possible.
> - Repeat three to five times (roughly, can be more if needed) before coming back to more controlled breathing. Whether that's nasal or mouth is up to you, and it depends on the context to which you are running in.

Don't always dump!

The main thing you're going to get an immediate benefit from is the carbon dioxide dump. I'm not going to lie, it feels good when you get it right. But it comes with a caution! If you are always dumping carbon dioxide, you're not building up your tolerance to it. Something I was horrified to find out with an elite athlete I'd worked with. I'd taught the carbon dioxide dump in one session, with strict instructions to use it sparingly, which he nodded along to. I then didn't see him again for about a month. At the next session, when I asked how the breath training had been, he replied, 'Brilliant, Jacko, loving those carbon dioxide dumps, doing them all the time, mate!' *What part of don't use them all the time, or you're not building up your tolerance didn't he understand?* A lesson learned for me with my coaching; it's a point to overemphasise, hence this overexaggerated explanation. I don't want you to make the same mistake.

That said, the carbon dioxide dump is so effective that the athlete felt the difference in his high-intensity training so much that he wanted to use it all the time. Depending on your training schedule, it's likely that most of your training isn't at so high an intensity you'll need to use it. But it's helpful for interval training, fartlek sessions, hill sprints, etc. Just don't overuse it. Use it at the right time, in the right context for the specific purpose of regaining control.

Putting it into practice

For your next run, don't start off mouth breathing if the intensity at the start and in the warm-up allows you to nasal breathe. Use that time to practise nasal breathing, training your diaphragm and regulating the speed of your breathing to allow you to relax into the run. If the pace and intensity increase so you can't ventilate enough with your nose, before it gets too uncomfortable, open your mouth. Not wide to start with, just a bit – use your mouth like a nose.

If you're picking up the pace further, doing some intervals or repeat sprints or just hit a steep hill on a run, remember our new hack! Try the CO_2 dump to get rid of some excess carbon dioxide to help you stay in control of your breathing rate.

We knew before we started there would be times when we need to use our mouth, but we want to ensure we are using it effectively and efficiently rather than slipping back to old compensatory habits of fast, shallow panting. Earning the right to mouth breathe is a process rather than a compensation; it takes time to change the auto and our diaphragm is key to that. I said we'd learn some tools to help us improve our mouth breathing along that journey, whether it's using the mouth like a nose, syncing the active exhales with our foot strikes or dumping off carbon dioxide. Tools in your locker to help you use your mouth most effectively when your nose just isn't enough. Regardless of which hole in your face you're using to get air in and out, remember, always using your diaphragm is one of the most important fundamentals.

Key takeaways

- Depending on the intensity you're running at, and the size of your nose and level of adaptation to nasal breathing, you might need to use your mouth to oxygenate your muscles sufficiently.
- The natural urge to mouth breathe is to adopt faster, shallower breathing, which is inefficient.
- Make your mouth work like a nose. A small gap provides some level of airflow resistance that can help slow down your breathing and engage your diaphragm when mouth breathing, keeping breathing more efficient.
- When you are really at your limit, use a few carbon dioxide dumps as a hack to get back control of your breathing.

I was introduced to Jacko after some our players and Premiership Clubs started to utilise his skillsets while out of camp. Over the past few seasons, we have brought Jacko into camp to both educate staff and to work with our players to great effect. We've had some great discussions around the role and effects of breathwork on movement, health and well-being and how we can develop this further for our players' benefit; from up- and down-regulation of the nervous system to enhancing movement efficiency, from enhancing sleep quality to reducing perceived threat.

All these things matter to us. Increasing numbers of our athletes are now utilising the benefits of his philosophy to prepare themselves physically, mentally and emotionally for the demands of international rugby and we look forward to continuing our relationship.

Bob Stewart, England Rugby medical lead senior men's team

CHAPTER 12

Recovery is a skill

Breathing is an essential part of improving recovery and, just like breathing, recovery is a skill. You're about to learn the power your breath has over your nervous system. It will help improve both recovery during (intra) and after (post) training. We'll even challenge ourselves to create adaptations so that the harder you train, the quicker you can recover.

What a difference a year makes

It was 5:55 a.m. on Sunday morning, the sun was just starting to rise. It was still dark down at base camp. I was approaching the final part of my seventh lap of 10-mile loops since yesterday morning. I was deep into a 24-hour mountain race, where each 10-mile lap amassed nearly 1000m of elevation. With just over four hours left in this 24-hour event, the marshal asked me if I was stopping like the majority of the other runners coming into the turnaround checkpoint. I shouted, 'F*ck no, I'm here for eight laps and we've got four hours left, I'm straight back out.'

However, their doubt made me doubt . . . but I came straight back to the plan. The plan was to start the final lap (lap eight) at 6:30 a.m., so I was 30 minutes ahead of schedule. The plan said we could do it. I followed the plan.

The plan of eight laps required me to cover 80 miles with nearly 8000m of elevation in under 24 hours. It was the plan because I only managed six laps the year before in 2023 when the winner achieved an incredible eight. My competitive nature – wanting to mix it with the big boys at the front – meant I was back this year for eight laps. It was an ambitious 33% improvement, and as a relative newbie to ultra-running, I didn't really have any right to be mixing it with the front runners. But with the plan in place, fuelled by the power of my breath, I managed it. I achieved 33% more in 2024; I was less fatigued, recovered faster and felt so much better even though I never stopped. Despite all that, I still didn't mix it with the front runners – they moved the goal posts without telling me, as a number of runners hit a staggering nine laps in total (which I thought was impossible after last year). I came in ninth place and couldn't have been happier. At the time I put that down as the best physical and mental performance of my life. *What made the biggest difference?* I managed my nervous system. *How did I do it?* Through my breath, of course!

One of the most powerful and immediate effects your breathing can have on your performance is the impact on recovery. Breathing is the remote control of the ANS. Your breathing directly impacts your heart rate, and exercise physiologists use heart rate as a key indicator of recovery. You'll notice you can get your breathing back under control, yet your heart rate will stay elevated for longer. But once you have your breathing under control, you can control and regulate your heart rate with your breath. If you know how.

What did this look like for me during an 80-mile ultra-marathon, running up and down a more-than-1000m mountain eight times? During the 8000m of ascents, it looked like trying to be as efficient with my breathing as possible. On the descents though, they were not just easier and an opportunity to run faster – I saw them as an opportunity to recover. A chance to calm breathing and calm the nervous system. This was a 24-hour race; it was about preserving energy and keeping going. Yes, it was a race against the clock, but I broke it down to individual reps that have a 'hard work' section on the way up and a 'recovery period' on the way down. I came down far faster than I went up, but the focus was on using the breathing to down-regulate my ANS, reduce sympathetic stress and lower my heart rate. So, when I came down into base camp for the checkpoint and turnaround, subjectively I felt better because my physiology was in a better state. Heart rate was lower, sympathetic stress lower and I'd recovered enough to go again.

I grabbed some food and drink from Catherine at the checkpoint and kept heading straight back out. You can think about it as a massive set of hill sprints. As you do hill sprints or hill runs, you work hard on the way up, your breathing might be really challenged, and then your rest and recovery period is typically the walk or gentle jog back down the hill. If you allow your breathing to be on auto and you're panting quickly as you walk back down the hill for your recovery, you don't regain control of your breathing as fast. Your heart rate at the start of the next hill sprint rep will be higher than if you controlled your breathing to regulate your heart rate.

As a direct comparison, when I managed 'only' six laps the year before, the third of those six reps was at an average pace of 11:13min/km with a heart rate of 142bpm. Comparatively, in 2024, when I managed eight laps, my fifth lap was at a comparable pace of 11:16min/km and my heart rate was only 133bpm, nearly 10bpm less on average than the year before, as well as the fact it was my fifth lap and not my third!

Why doesn't your body do this automatically when you're trying to recover? Remember, just because breathing is automatic, doesn't mean it's optimal. Your body doesn't want you to go and run up a big mountain again, climbing over 1000m in a 10-mile loop in two to three hours. So, it doesn't automatically breathe in a way that facilitates good recovery, so you feel good enough to want to go again. Going again would be more stress, and your brain is trying to preserve itself and, ultimately, seek safety. We have to do something intentionally different with our breathing if we want to push our limits and discover what we are truly capable of.

Importance of regulating heart rate

That story was an example of using breathing to help recovery during running, as well as how to use breathing to down-regulate the nervous system. Due to the extreme nature of that 24-hour event, I was doing both within the same event. But typically, down-regulation is done post training. It separates recovery into two distinct phases that we will look at individually: intra (during) recovery breathing and post (after) recovery breathing.

Yet there is something linking those two separate recovery processes: the effect that breathing has on your heart rate. Before we start looking at intra-recovery breathing, let's first explain why.

Our breathing and heart rate are interwoven and intimately linked within our ANS. They communicate with one another; when we are well regulated, that communication is clearer. With every breath we take (which is hard to say without singing), our heart rate speeds up on the inhale. With every exhale, the heart rate slows down. If we are able to extend the time period of the exhale compared with the inhale, we can increase the time spent in the second half of the breathing cycle, which affects heart rate reduction.

Dr Andy Galpin, a professor of kinesiology, is an advocate of using heart rate as a key indicator of cardiovascular fitness and ability to recover. His belief is the faster someone can regulate their heart rate immediately post training session, the better their recovery. Dr Galpin explains that those in a training block who recover their heart rate quicker make more performance progress within a training block due to improved recovery compared with someone who takes longer to regulate their heart rate back down to baseline. We're about to learn how to do it better.

Intra-recovery breathing

Research has shown that how we breathe can affect how well our heart rate recovers during running sessions.[1] It's not just as simple as 'slow down your exhales', and there are a couple of key points to help us use our breathing to recover better.

First, slowing exhales can be difficult when you are feeling out of breath at the end of a run or between interval sets for a number of reasons. If you're mechanically challenged by ribcage alignment, tightness in the ribcage or function of your diaphragm, it will affect your ability to ventilate during the inhale, which dictates how much air you have to exhale. When you have a smaller volume of air to exhale, it makes it harder to slow it down.

Second, during the exhale when you're feeling out of breath, your brain is trying to offload the larger amounts of carbon dioxide. Your chemosensitivity in the respiratory centres of the brain will affect how comfortable you are at slowing down the rate of carbon dioxide leaving the lungs as you try to control those exhales. Your psychological response to the feeling of being out of breath will also affect your ability to control it. The higher your carbon dioxide tolerance, the more comfortable you are with the perception of air hunger, and the more you practise recovery as a skill, the easier it is to control and slow your exhale.

A slight warning. It's a bit of a 'Goldilocks' situation with exhales. If you control them too much, you can make yourself feel even more out of breath. There's a sweet spot where you're in control of the exhale without overly slowing it down. You can make dramatic changes to how fast you recover and how much better you feel. Recovery is a skill, so it takes a little bit of practice. Like any skill, the more you practise it correctly, the better you get.

Effect of ribcage on breathing recovery

To use your breathing effectively to regulate and control your heart rate, it's helpful to have everything mechanically set up in your favour to optimise both inhalation and exhalation. The exhales are important for the regulation of your heart rate, and the inhales are important for the volume of air you ventilate, which dictates the volume of air you have to exhale. The more air you have to exhale, the easier it is to control it.

Your ability to mechanically ventilate, as we learned in chapter 8, is affected by the function of your diaphragm and the expansion of your ribcage. The alignment of your ribcage being vital in both. A 2019 study measured heart rate recovery between running intervals, tidal volume and end tidal carbon dioxide, which is the amount of carbon dioxide exhaled.[2] The study noted that our standing posture and position of the ribcage influenced the size of inhalation (tidal volume), amount of carbon dioxide that can be exhaled and how quickly the heart rate slows down.

If the ribcage is out of alignment and not stacked, we know this affects the position of the diaphragm and its ZOA, restricting the diaphragm and reducing tidal volume. When we're more 'stacked', with the ribcage aligned with the pelvis, the diaphragm functions better. The result is a larger tidal volume, carbon dioxide expired at a faster rate – as the exhale is also bigger when the inhale is bigger, so regaining breath control is easier – helping heart rate reduce quicker.

TRY THIS

- Put your hands on your head, let your back arch and pelvis tilt forwards and try to take a big breath in – you'll feel restricted.
- Compare that with leaning forwards and putting your hands on your knees – notice that you can relax your stomach as you support yourself – and then take a big breath in.
- That breath will feel bigger in size and your diaphragm easier to use more fully.

You can also test the difference lying down when you are even more supported to see the effect the position of your ribcage has on your ability to ventilate larger volumes of air.

- Lying completely flat with legs straight out, arch your back, let your pelvis roll forwards and push your ribcage up towards the ceiling.
- With ribcage pushed up and your back arched as much as you can, try and take a deep inhale. You're restricted.
- Now compare that with the semi-supine position (from chapter 8) with your ribcage nicely stacked and aligned with your pelvis.
- Now take a full and deep inhalation – I bet that feels massive in comparison.

The position of the ribcage is key to the position and function of the diaphragm. Even if you're supported by the floor, if the ribcage is out of alignment, your diaphragm is compromised and therefore inhalation is restricted. Likewise, if your ribcage is tight, and your diaphragm jacked up and restricted, it's going to be harder to increase your tidal volume regardless of your posture – hence the emphasis on using my breathing mobilisations and diaphragm exercises.

Exercise: Breathing recovery 'in sessions' (Intra)

It might have come as a bit of a surprise that rather than focusing on the inhale (although still important), the focus of this intra-recovery protocol is more about the exhalation. We think we need more oxygen, but it's actually the exhale that is key. Scientist Xavier Woorons showed us that reoxygenation of muscle tissue is more to do with what you do in training rather than how you take your first few inhales during your recovery period.

Despite the exhale being key, that doesn't mean the inhale isn't important. Of course, it is. A good exhale starts at the end of a good inhale. A full inhale also helps to stimulate those mechanoreceptors in the diaphragm and lungs that reduce the sensation of air hunger. Plus, we've learned that the volume of carbon dioxide we can offload in our exhalation is dictated by the volume of our inhale.

How do most people breathe when they are out of breath? Short, fast, shallow breaths into the upper chest. We're not going to let that compensatory habit stop us from recovering quicker – no! We are going to learn to optimise our breathing recovery. Just like Olympic 400m runner Iwan Thomas explained to me during his hardest training sessions when 'swimming in lactate', how he was filling his lungs was key to how well he recovered.

IRBP: Intra-recovery breathing protocol

Intra-recovery breathing refers to how we optimise our breathing during training and running sessions to regulate breathing rate and heart rate. This intra-recovery breathing protocol (IRBP) is something I coach all the elite athletes I work with, and it is particularly beneficial during higher-intensity sessions, such as interval training.

> **EXERCISE: INTRA-RECOVERY BREATHING PROTOCOL**
> - Alignment of ribcage to optimise diaphragm function is key.
> - Stand tall, big chest, ribs back with ribcage stacked on top of pelvis, and show me your poker face – body language is important!
> - Take a large volume of air on the inhale using your diaphragm and ribcage expansion fully, and stimulate those stretch receptors in your diaphragm and lungs to help reduce sensation of being out of breath.
> - Filling from the bottom up, expand your ribcage 360 degrees as the diaphragm moves down to the pelvis like a pump and your lower ribs move upwards and outwards.
> - Get control of the exhale, but not too much. Make it gradual and find that 'just right' Goldilocks sweet spot.
> - Get back to nasal breathing gradually. You might have needed to use your mouth at the start of the process, depending on how out of breath you felt.
> - Gradually extend your exhale when it feels comfortable to do so.
> - Finally, as you extend your exhales gradually, allow the size and volume of the inhale to gradually reduce as you feel calmer.

At the beginning, if you feel like you can't start the process because you feel so out of breath, incorporate the carbon dioxide dumps we outlined in the last chapter. Offload a large amount of carbon dioxide as quickly and efficiently as possible using the mouth, allowing you to start the IRBP, even during the hardest of interval sessions.

A great example of this was with Ollie Marchon, who took on the Trans Alpine Trail in 2024 – a beautiful but brutal week-long mountain ultra-race in the Alps. He'd never done anything like this before. We did some work together to help with his breathing during preparation for such a gruelling event. As part of his preparation, we did a training run together where we managed a marathon in the mountains, amassing nearly 3000m of elevation as we summited Yr Wyddfa (Snowdon) – not just for his first-ever time but twice more. Yes, we climbed that bad boy three times during a 40km training run. This was what just one day looked like as part of the Trans Alpine race, which lasted an entire week.

Seven days back-to-back in the Alps was going to push his limits, so recovery was going to be a key focus. We did some specific work over a couple of sessions on the efficiency of his breathing mechanics, his ability to regulate his breathing rate and the effect it would have on his heart rate recovery. After completing the Trans Alpine Trail he said, 'It was helpful to regulate recovery with nasal breathing at the top of the climbs to help regulate my heart rate.' Getting back to nasal breathing and controlling his breathing rate helped Ollie regulate his heart rate better between each of the brutal climbs.

Post-recovery breathing

The key to post training or competition recovery is the ability to control the ANS with your breathing to down-regulate. Our breathing is the gateway to the nervous system. Rather than just trying to regulate the heart rate before the next rep in an interval session, we want to switch the system from being sympathetically dominated (fight or flight) to parasympathetically active (rest, digest and recovery) once the session, competition or day (in a multi-day ultra) is over. We need to be able to down-regulate the entire system. It's our breathing that can make the switch.

The link between your breathing and your parasympathetic nervous system is your vagus nerve. Simplistically, HRV (Heart Rate Variability) – which those of you with wearable technology can get biofeedback for – can be thought of as a measure of vagus nerve health and parasympathetic tone, although in reality, it's far more complex than that. Your vagus nerve sends information back to your brain, providing vital feedback about what is most important at that time. Where are the body's resources needed? When training, you need sympathetic activation that drives blood flow to your working muscles and increases heart rate and focus. But you don't want or need that once you have finished your session. After your session, the importance needs to be on repair and recovery. But our brain needs to feel safe to switch resources towards that mode. Many of us will go from the physical stress of a training run, to the mental stress of a busy job or simply our lives, which can easily feel stressful and overwhelming. Even though you've stopped the physical stress of running, your nervous system will stay in a state of sympathetic activation unless the system feels safe enough to shut down some of the fight or flight response. The vagus nerve provides the communication, and your breathing is a great way to show some love to that vagus nerve, helping to promote better recovery and sleep.[3]

De-stress with down-regulation

In his book *Out of Thin Air*, runner and author Michael Crawley noted when living and training with elite Ethiopian runners, in comparison to them, 'We aren't great at resting, we don't know how to relax.'[4] He noted that one of the things that appeared to separate the best runners was their ability to adapt and recover. They take recovery very seriously. They sleep between sessions and try to reduce physical output away from training as much as possible. They know how to relax and switch off. In contrast, many of us recreational runners are probably stressed from work and life and don't know how to switch off and relax. And as Dr Martin Yelling explained, if you carry that stress into your running, it's going to be very hard to find the relaxation needed for fluid and efficient running. Many of the conversations I have with medics, physiotherapists and support staff for elite athletes is that day to day, the athletes are too stressed, finding it difficult to switch off, which affects muscle tone, sleep, recovery and even injuries.

Having worked with elite and international athletes and teams, I agree with Crawley and observe we're not really providing tools that actually work at the nervous system level when we talk about aiding recovery for athletes. At best, we focus on things that help reduce musculoskeletal aches and pains, such as massage, stretching, etc. At worst, we do no cool down and nothing recovery focused as part of our training schedule. Other gadgets and gizmos have become popular, such as red-light therapy, vibration massage tools, ice baths, saunas and compression garments. I don't have a problem with any of those things; I have used most of them. But none of them work deeply on the ANS as breathing does because none of them are woven into the ANS in the way that breathing is.

I remember doing some research about a decade ago about recovery for the athletes I was supporting as a strength and conditioning coach, before I'd learned anything about breathing. One study from 2009 concluded that, 'The perceived effectiveness of recovery modalities was commonly reported to be impacted by the athletes' and/or coaches' feelings as a result of general observations, past experiences, and instinct.'[5] It therefore highlighted the importance of how you feel about a recovery protocol, even if others might rightly or wrongly label it as a placebo. If you felt better afterwards, it was worth doing. Which reminds me of the quote from Dr Alia Crum, an associate professor of psychology at Stanford University: 'The total effect of anything is a combined product of what you're doing and what you think about what you're doing.' What I see now is that whatever recovery strategy you choose to adopt, you are going to be breathing when using it. How you breathe has the power to shift your ANS to a state of rest, repair and recovery. So why not use both?

Exercise: Post-recovery – Calm breathing = calm nervous system

A number of breathing-related modalities have been shown to help stimulate that important vagus nerve to aid the recovery process: slower breathing, deeper breathing using the diaphragm fully, longer exhales and humming.[6] When we calm our breathing, we calm our nervous system.

My favourite tool for promoting recovery and down-regulating the ANS is humming exhales. Humming innovates the vagus and down-regulates the nervous system. That's because the vibrations that humming creates help to stimulate the vagus nerve as it passes through the voice box. The process of humming also helps to slow down and extend our exhales, which helps slow heart rate and promote parasympathetic activity. Humming does it naturally – you don't need to put any effort in, you simply relax and follow this process:

PRBP: Post-recovery breathing protocol

Post-run or session recovery is all about the nervous system and the relationship between our exhales and the relaxation response. So, a comfortable lying position where you can fully relax is beneficial for this one.

> ### EXERCISE: PRBP
>
> *A full video tutorial of the following exercise can be found online at www.thebreathrunningcoach.com/recovery-breathing*
>
>
>
> - Before starting, I like to take my current resting breathing rate, so time 30 seconds and count your breathing (as per the assessment in chapter 7, so we can compare at the end).
> - Start lying down so you can fully relax in a comfortable position. If you need to support your neck, have a small cushion or pillow behind your head.
> - If you are doing this immediately after finishing a training session, you may still feel a little out of breath and your heart rate may still be higher. Take a few fuller, larger and deeper breaths initially, using the larger volume of air on the inhale to help you start to slow the exhale down so you feel less out of breath.
> - Put your tongue on the roof of your mouth, mouth closed, lips softly together, jaw relaxed and allow your breathing to naturally settle.
> - Inhale through (not up) your nose, following your airflow to the back of your throat, noticing the sensation of air in the airway and any sound your breath is making.
> - Choose to make your breath quieter as you inhale and soften the sensation of airflow in the airway.
> - Notice that as you soften your airflow and make your breath gradually silent, the speed of your breathing naturally slows down and becomes calmer. →

- We will shift more into a parasympathetic state by extending our exhales and stimulating the vagus nerve with humming.
- On your next exhale, with the jaw relaxed, mouth closed and lips together, make a humming noise as you naturally extend the exhale.
- The vibrations of the humming innervate the vagus nerve where it passes through your voice box.
- Keep your inhales relaxed, calm and silent.
- As you continue humming and your exhales become longer, allow yourself to keep relaxing.

Continue with the humming exhales for a few minutes until you feel completely relaxed. Have a swallow and observe the increase in saliva in the mouth as the body shifts in parasympathetic tone (rest, digest). That's the relaxation response, and the saliva is a physical sign that you're doing it.

Notice how relaxed and calm your breathing is. Notice how calm and relaxed your body feels. You might even feel like your body has sunk into the floor. When you are ready, you can time 30 seconds again, as you did at the start, and count your breathing to see how your natural respiratory rate has changed.

With a bit of practice, many of you will now only take three or so breaths in 30 seconds, as your breathing rate during the humming has likely reduced to around six breaths per minute. This has been shown to be an effective breathing rate to improve HRV – a biological marker of recovery.

This might just be the single best thing you will do with your breathing to help improve your physical and mental state. It feels nice to be relaxed and breathing calmly, doesn't it?

Breathing works!

Both intra- and post-recovery breathing can be absolute game changers. It's one of the biggest things I wish I'd known when I played professional rugby: that there is something you can actually do that is totally in your control, to help you feel less out of breath and bring your heart rate down.

A great example of how effective this can be in just one training session was with a female recreational runner who reduced her heart rate recovery time by over 170% when implementing the IRBP.

A more extreme example of this is in contact sports like rugby where the intensity is high and recovery periods are short, so we have almost no time at all to catch the breath and reset. The players need to be very quick and efficient at regulating. Professional Super League player Ollie Partington found it helpful for his recovery. 'I love it, I can regulate back to baseline quicker in any session now,' he stated, having practised and integrated the recovery tools into his training over an entire season.

Sometimes the down-regulation is so powerful it's the only thing I work on with an athlete. None of the breath-holds, none of the NT, just purely the regulation of their nervous system post training to help with recovery and enhance sleep – it's a game changer on its own. If you only do one thing, do this.

I'll never forget the text message and screenshot I received from an international athlete who started wearing their WHOOP band again after starting to follow the post-recovery breathing protocol (PRBP). The recovery scores relating to HRV were always around 80% at best. The week they started following the down-regulation breathing protocol after training or before bed, the score jumped up into the 90s. By the end of the week, I got a text with a screenshot from their WHOOP showing a 100% recovery score, which they said they'd never had and they were totally shocked. 'Breathing works,' I replied!

Putting it into practice

At the heart of getting better and becoming a stronger runner is becoming better at recovery. When putting this into practice, it's important to ask and understand a key question: Do I want to make recovery easier in the immediate term or do I want to challenge myself to make longer-term adaptations?

You need two very different approaches when answering yes to either. Some people will potentially miss a very important point with this.

You might be thinking, *Well, Jacko, I always want to make recovery as easy or as fast as possible!* But that might not always be the case; let me explain.

In a competition or a race then, yes, you want to maximise everything at your disposal to improve your performance, reduce fatigue and enhance recovery. This may also be the case during a higher-intensity interval session or hill sprint session. But there are times in training when you actually want to make recovery tougher or harder to create a stimulus that invokes an adaptation over time. It's essentially what all 'training' is, but for some reason we forget about this with recovery.

Using your nose in a recovery period rather than your mouth is a great way to train the contractile strength of your diaphragm and associated inspiratory muscles. It might feel harder than using your mouth – it essentially is – but that's good because it's like a 'strength' training session for your diaphragm. The resistance from the nose also slows down the air as it's leaving your lungs. That means you automatically get some practice of a key component in slowing down your exhales, which is both a skill and requires some physiological adaptations. As the exhaled air is leaving the lungs more slowly you will be retaining more carbon dioxide than your body and the chemoreceptors in your brain are used to, helping improve your carbon dioxide tolerance.

That means you are creating a 'training adaptation' even during your recovery periods. In order to create that adaptation you need the stimulus which might feel a bit 'harder' and not 'natural' at the start. But that's the purpose of training, and you'll become a stronger runner who recovers better.

The more you practise the skill of using your breathing to regulate your heart rate and recovery, the better you get at doing it. You've now got tools that give you direct access to your nervous system. When you consciously choose to control your breathing, you control your nervous system, heart rate and recovery. Your ability to use them is a result of practice and the adaptations you've created through the techniques you've learned.

Nothing is in isolation; we are always breathing, and we can optimise recovery with our breathing regardless of any other recovery protocol you like to use. When you recover better, you can relax in a training session, which helps with running performance in the short term. In the long term, when you recover better, you sleep better. When you sleep better, you wake up ready to perform at a higher level, and you build resilience to the stresses of life and your training. That's the magic in recovery and it's hidden in our breath.

Key takeaways

- There are two great opportunities to use breathing for recovery: during (intra) running sessions to lower the heart rate and regulate breathing rate and after (post) training to down-regulate the nervous system, promoting improved recovery and sleep.
- Recovery is a skill. The more you practise controlling your breathing and heart rate in a session, the better you get at it. It's the same with your down-regulation – you get better at controlling your nervous system.
- Recovery and regulation start even before the session or run is finished, meaning you can be better regulated and less stressed (more relaxed) during the session or you can run knowing you've regulated your breathing.

Since working on my breathing with Jacko my sleep has improved, my recovery is better, and I can get back in control of my breathing and regulate faster than anyone else on the pitch, which gives me a huge competitive advantage.

Henry Arundell, England Rugby

CHAPTER 13

Integrating into training and races

It's about to get even more exciting as we put things into practice, learning how to integrate these breathing techniques into our running. We'll look at some important nuances to understand the difference between what to do in training sessions and races, covering everything from 5km to ultra-marathons.

The Norwegian 4×4 method

Every time I open up my YouTube, I'm bombarded with videos about the 4×4 Norwegian method. It was developed by exercise physiologist Dr Jan Hoff and made famous by Jakob Ingebrigtsen, who won gold medals at Tokyo and Paris Olympics in the 1500m and 5000m, respectively. I loved the collaboration of sports science and the proof in the pudding when Ingebrigtsen took gold on the biggest of stages.

The 4×4 Norwegian method is a brutal form of interval training designed to take your VO_2 max, lactate threshold and tolerance to epic levels. It involves running for four minutes at around 85% to 95% of your maximum heart rate. You get three minutes of rest before going again for another four minutes. You do these a brutal four times, hence the 4×4.

I wanted to try it out. I wanted to feel the lactate building in my legs and how my breathing would respond to the intense four minutes of 85–95% max heart rate with only three minutes of rest between four bouts of those four-minute efforts.

I knew it was going to be tough, so I tried to find the flattest 1.5km near my house – which is impossible – to avoid making the four minutes more brutal than they needed to be by adding unnecessarily hills within a rep. I like challenging myself in training and pushing the limits of not just the body but also the mind, but adding hill reps into the 4×4 method would be not only stupid but likely detrimental to the adaptations we're trying to achieve with this session.

I completed a short warm-up, made sure my watch was tracking, time, distance and my heart. I was armed with a number of breathing techniques to deploy during different parts of the session, and I wanted to track my heart rate to ensure I knew the effect my breathing techniques were having.

I flew out of the imaginary blocks as I sprinted down the street in my village, where I'm locally known as 'mad Dave' from my various training exploits (at least that's what I hope it's for!). For the first minute or so I was breathing nasally and gradually syncing my inhale with three strides and my exhale for four. Things started getting tasty pretty quickly, and I deployed turtle power to help ventilate up to 26% more air through my nose. As I passed through two minutes, I felt like I couldn't maintain this intensity breathing nasally anymore and made the switch to mouth breathing. Mouth only slightly open, so I still had a small amount of resistance, but I was aware that I was still using my diaphragm. It was hard, but I felt in control of my breathing, even though it was being challenged, and I could maintain some degree of that important relaxation.

Four minutes was up as I reached the cattle grid that signalled the other end of the village. My heart rate was sky high, reaching 180bpm, which for a 42-year-old is beyond my theoretical max. I dumped carbon dioxide like it was going out of fashion, which allowed me to get back in control of my breathing relatively quickly. I got back to nasal breathing and gradually started to slow my heart rate, trusting the IRBP. After two minutes I felt pretty good and looked down at my watch. My heart rate was right back down at 100 with still another minute before I had to go again.

It's a great example of leaning into different breathing techniques at various points in the session to optimise my performance or at least manage the brutality of these threshold sessions. It was tough and painful, but in all honesty, I actually really enjoyed the process. I think having breathing techniques to use took my mind off the brutal nature of the session. I wasn't wishing the session away, hoping it would be over quickly. No, I was keen to see how quickly I could get my heart rate down in the recovery and see how hard I could push it in the efforts and still maintain control of my diaphragmatic breathing.

I took on the Norwegian 4×4 method and came out the other side with Jacko's 'Norwegian breathing method'!

Optimise or adaptation?

In an event or race, you are trying to optimise efficiency and relaxation as much as possible. In your training runs, you're honing breathing efficiency, which requires you to provide a stimulus to force that adaptation. In training it's not always about making breathing easier if you want to improve. If you want the diaphragm to increase in strength and endurance, you've got to make it work harder. If you want to increase your carbon dioxide tolerance and ventilatory threshold, you need to spend some time exposed to higher levels of carbon dioxide and lactate. We can use the various different breathing techniques we've covered thus far to do exactly that.

SAID principle

Specific adaptation to imposed demands – the SAID principle – is one of the first principles of training we get taught in strength and conditioning education. In simple terms, it's a case of 'you get what you train for'. A really obvious example being that if you want to get better at nasal breathing when running but do all your running with your mouth open, you're not going to see the improvements you want. It's a silly example, but silly examples help make the point.

It's a principle I've always come back to no matter what the training is. It's simple, rational and effective in helping shape the choices of what we do in different training scenarios based on the purpose of the session. It's a principle that you can easily apply to your breath training when integrating into your running.

To make best use of the SAID principle, you need to understand the type of session you are doing, know the purpose of the session and what the adaptation you are trying to create is. Then select the method of breathing to help you achieve that purpose. Use the best breathing techniques at your disposal to optimise the stimulus and the forthcoming adaptations to recovery. Next are some simple, broader examples of applying the SAID principle, before we get into the specifics of how to use the breath-training tools outlined in different types of training sessions, events and races.

Asking yourself these two questions is helpful in making informed choices about which breathing techniques will help you optimise each training session:

- Is the session aerobic or anaerobic in nature?
- Do I want to make recovery as easy and quick as possible for short-term benefit or am I looking to challenge the recovery for longer-term adaptations?

If the session is aerobic, then we want to be using oxygen as efficiently as possible and, in that scenario, we'll look at how nasal breathing is helpful for both pacing and honing aerobic efficiency with zone 2 training, as an example. If the session is anaerobic, intervals perhaps, then we are looking to push our limits and use techniques that allow us to do that with our breathing. Shortening our step-to-breath ratio (SBR), active exhales and using the mouth like a nose are all things we might use to help us push our limits. We may also use CO_2 dumps in recovery periods during anaerobic sessions to help us regulate our breathing and heart rate as quickly as possible, yet in other recovery periods, we may choose nasal breathing as a challenge to our recovery process.

We'll look at race- and event-day tactics and how this differs from training in some situations. We'll see how different types of races and events may differ with individuals, but we'll start with some more specific training scenarios first.

Warm-ups

As runners, how often does our warm-up start with putting our trainers on and finish as we close the door behind us? Maybe not all of us, all the time, but, be honest, we are bad at warming up. More often than not, it never even enters our minds, let alone us actually doing anything physically to prepare our muscles, heart rate and breathing for what's ahead.

My hope is this can change, and being in control of your breathing can ignite that change. One thing I always programme into the start of athletes' warm-ups is the ribcage mobilisation exercises from chapter 9. They are great to open up the thoracic spine, hips and shoulders, as well as engaging the diaphragm and activating all the inhalation and exhalation musculature. It's like a breathing warm-up. If you've never done them prior to your normal warm-up or run, then it's a total game changer. 'Breathing feels easier' is the surprised comment most runners give me after we do them. When we measure their ventilation, they have increased their tidal volume, which helps them regulate a more efficient rate of breathing and stay more relaxed on the run.

The other key tool that's simple to integrate into warm-ups, when the intensity or pace is relatively low, is nasal breathing. This helps physiological and psychological regulation. Whether it's to help manage nerves and/or anxiety or to help 'dial in' and focus, many different types of runners have reported that integrating nasal breathing into the early parts of their warm-up is beneficial. Richard Whitehead, for example, described his breathing as a 'superpower' and explained, 'In my warm-ups I use breathing to help me focus and reduce tension. It's like a meditation. In the first 10 minutes I'm focused on nasal breathing as it helps me unlock the depth of breath. That's always part of my warm-up process for a run.'

The notion of starting slowly and using nasal breathing as a way to focus, guide a gradual warm-up pace and enhance relaxation was noted by Michael Crawley. In *Out of Thin Air* he observed the best Ethiopian runners and how slow and relaxed their warm-up pace was, just a 6 or 7min/km pace, allowing them to breathe with their nose and be relaxed, writing one of the runners was, 'so serene at this pace, he's breathing through his nose'.[1]

Start your run slowly (let your nose dictate the pace) and grab some nasal breathing benefits while the pace is easy. Get focused yet relaxed with the superpower of your breath.

Aerobic training runs

Easy runs: The 80/20 rule – Easy means easy

The latest research shows that nasal breathing is not only just possible to around 80–85% of our VO_2 max, but it's also more beneficial. It improves ventilatory efficiency, slows down our breathing, engages the diaphragm and helps us relax, when we can sufficiently ventilate enough air for the given pace.[2]

How much of your running training is meant to be above that type of 'threshold'? Shane Benzie told me, 'pretty much all running plans follow a simple 80/20 rule principle', something Dr Peter Attia, a physician and researcher, speaks regularly about, with 80% of our training being 'easy pace' in zone 2. Your zone 2 heart rate is hopefully well below 85% of your VO_2 max (it's typically quoted as around 60–70% of your VO_2 max). Most of your training could be done breathing nasally as a runner. It might even help keep you within your zone 2 training and not go too fast on your 'easy' runs.

Aerobic zone 2 training is at an all-time high in terms of popularity due to the likes of Dr Peter Attia drawing attention to it, for health and longevity benefits. If you need any more convincing, an interview in *Runner's World* magazine stated that around 80% of

Kipchoge's running sessions were said to be at an easy pace in zones 1 and 2 (but for him it's not that slow – it's between 4 and 5min/km).[3] The notion of running slowly to improve seems to be a bit of a paradox that most amateur runners fail to buy into fully. One of the biggest criticisms I've heard from running coaches is that amateur runners run too fast and too often relative to their ability. A friend of mine, who's now a sub-3-hour marathon runner, said that they thought every session needed to be hard to improve. Since learning that long 'easy' runs are actually meant to be easy, their marathon times got faster.

Nasal breathing can be a great way to hone breathing efficiency and manage pacing so those easy zone 2 runs actually stay in zone 2. This helps you benefit from the aerobic improvements in capillary, myoglobin and mitochondria development from aerobic training.[4]

When you ask yourself whether it is an aerobic or anaerobic session and you answer aerobic, choose to use the smaller holes in your face.

Controlling pace with step-to-breath ratios (SBRs)

As well as opening the door more easily to relaxation and a blissful flow state in running, the research into LRC shows that it's a helpful tool in modulating not just breathing rate but also controlling pace.

You can use LRC to develop a SBR ratio to match the desired pace for your running. Running coach Jack Daniels explains that setting a SBR is especially helpful for pacing on easy zone 2 runs; it helps you understand how hard you're pushing yourself. Essentially, your breathing is a great feedback system if you understand what it's telling you, and, most importantly, if you listen to it.

Daniels's theory on this is backed up by the research in to LRC, which states that 'different LRC ratios could thus be utilized as a "gears" system corresponding to different perceptual and physiological levels of effort'.[5]

Which is exactly what I've developed. A system of SBRs that not only provide feedback regarding how much we're pushing but lets us set a pace more easily, stay more relaxed and access flow state, as well as track our progress. With me, for example, initially I'd enjoy and feel relaxed on easy runs with a three-step inhale and a four-step exhale at a 5:30min/km pace. With training and a combination of improved breathing and running form, my easy 5:30min/km pace is now with a four-step inhale and five-step exhale. Even though I'm going at the same pace, it feels easier and I'm breathing slower, which helps with relaxation, a slower heart rate and a reduced perception of effort.

Now, I'm not saying that a four-step inhale and five-step exhale is a magic formula that works for everyone. It's a ratio that I like for my easy runs, specific to me, my fitness levels, running ability and breath control. You need to experiment and find out what feels most relaxing and best for you. Try it out, play with it, experiment on yourself. Give it a chance – I wish I had done years ago, but when I first tried, I didn't like the prescriptive nature of it.

Like me, Anna Harding from 'The Running Channel' has experienced pain on her right side and heard that LRC and balancing out her foot strikes might help relieve the pain when running. She's done plenty of Pilates and knows how to breathe diaphragmatically, but like me, when she first tried LRC, she found it frustrating and gave up on it before it could work its magic.

It's true that some people don't like it initially, and it's important to say that some researchers noted test subjects found the instructions 'annoying', especially so in untrained runners.[6] It's not something you have to do. It's something to try, but don't dismiss it if at first you don't like it. Remember, the elites do it naturally, so with some training and practice you'll notice that you start to find a more economical rhythm without trying or even counting your steps. I know now, I can hit the four-step inhale and five-step exhale on my easy runs without counting steps. I've just trained it. My body likes it; it feels better and easier and so it just happens naturally now.

Let's look at three specific SBRs you can use as a starting point: easy 4:5, medium 3:4 and high 2:2 (but remember, you can experiment and tailor yourself).

Easy SBR 4:5
- Inhale for a count of four foot strikes.
- Exhale for a count of five foot strikes.

This easy ratio or 'low gear' is ideal for pacing our long easy runs. The total number of steps is nine for a full breath cycle. The odd number ensures that we're not always landing on the same foot at the end of the exhale, and hence my left foot doesn't hurt anymore!

During my VO_2 max testing, the exact point I couldn't comfortably manage a four-step inhale and five-step exhale with my nose was the point when lactate was just starting creeping up and I was about to transition into zone 3. If you are aware of your breathing, it can give you vital feedback not only about which zone you're in but also where you are within it. When using this SBR on an easy run where the aim is to stay in zone 2, if I ever start to feel like I've finished my exhale and run out of air before I've taken my fifth step, I know that I'm pushing my lactate up and moving out of zone 2, so I can back off and regulate my pace accordingly.

Now that, of course, doesn't mean it's the same for you, but it is very interesting to note that there appears to be a correlation between breathing and lactate. What's helpful to understand is what that felt like (unless you are going to have your own VO_2 max test and then you can check for yourself). The transition from zone 2 to 3 still felt comfortable, I didn't suddenly feel out of breath. I needed to go active on my inhales and consciously try to ventilate more air during that inhalation rather than it being relaxed and natural.

If you listen to your breathing, are aware of your nasal breathing on easy runs and receptive to your ventilation sensations, you'll soon be able to regulate your pace through your breathing and your SBR to keep you in zone 2 with pinpoint accuracy. Those long easy runs stop becoming boring long runs where you want to go faster. Instead they become a chance to hone the efficiency of your nasal breathing, breathing mechanics and diaphragm strength and enjoy the hypnotic meditative state that LRC seduces you into.

Medium SBR 3:4
- Inhale for a count of three foot strikes.
- Exhale for a count of four foot strikes.

The second ratio is medium, where during VO_2 max testing I was active on the inhale, initiating those stretch mechanoreceptors in the lungs to purposefully increase tidal volume. I counted three foot strikes as the size of my inhalation increased, and I ventilated more air at the required faster rate in order to oxygenate efficiently as my body desperately tried to keep lactate under control as we approached zone 4. The three-step inhales followed by four-step exhales created seven steps in total for one breath cycle, again an odd total number, meaning we're not landing on the same foot at the end of each exhale. This is the type of gear I would switch into during a climb (depending on how steep it is) or if I'm ready to push the pace a little bit on running longer intervals.

I've personally found this to be a great ratio to help push on my prolonged efforts either in longer interval sessions or on climbs in mountain races when I feel like I want to walk on a climb. When I focus on this ratio, I know I can maintain it. My Moxy near-infrared spectrometer shows that my muscle oxygen saturation levels remain stable when I maintain this ratio. It means that despite feeling like I want to walk on a climb, if I check-in with my SBR and I can manage to keep to 3:4, then I know I'm oxygenating sufficiently regardless of how tired I feel. It's surprising how much more of a climb I continue to run on with this in mind and helping pace the effort. Because the testing shows that I am oxygenating effectively, I can trust in it and ignore the perception of fatigue, which has other parameters affecting it, not just oxygen supply.

Specifically, as a percentage of VO_2 max and training zones, this ratio took me through zone 3 to the edge of zone 4. What took me into zone 4 towards zone 5 was using the same medium of SBR but stacking it with turtle power. With turtle power, my ventilation increased by 26% and, using the medium 3:4 ratio I was able to stay regulated with my breathing rate and perception of effort, as the VO_2 max test ramped up in intensity. I hit 87.5% of my VO_2 max before finally having to switch to mouth breathing and the high SBR as I entered zone 5.

High SBR 2:2

- Inhale for a count of two foot strikes.
- Exhale for a count of two foot strikes.

The high ratio is the point when you are pushing your limits towards the finish line, facing a really steep climb or are doing some hard threshold interval sessions. Rather than just emptying the tank, losing control of your breathing rate and volume – or worse, losing your relaxation and form – using the highest SBR can help you to stay relatively regulated as you push your limits.

In this gear I've gone beyond my NT (87.5% VO_2 max), where I can't ventilate enough air through my nose and have to use my mouth. Of course, regulating the speed of breath is helped by the step count, but you also want to make sure you've 'earned the right to mouth breathe'. The inhale is going to come relatively quickly in this gear, so you need to make sure your diaphragm is working well and you're not going to jump into shallow upper chest breathing as a compensation because you have your mouth open. Making the mouth work like a nose can help with this, as we discussed in chapter 11.

The high SBR is a two-step inhale and two-step exhale; Jack Daniels noticed that elite runners use it when pushing their limits. Although the total number of steps is an even number (four), meaning you'll land on the same foot repeatedly at the end of each exhale, this gear is not designed to be used for hours at a time. Use this gear when you need it, and you'll blow your opponents away. If you want an extra boost in this gear, a bit like a mushroom in Mario kart, synchronise your push offs on the exhale with strong forceful exhales from Breathplay – a secret weapon to keep up your sleeve!

One final tip with using LRC, start with the exhale rather than the inhale. For example, if you're using a 3:4 SBR as part of an interval session, at the start of each rep:

- Take a nice deep nasal inhalation so you have a decent volume of air in your lungs to control the exhale.
- Finish the inhale before you start running.

- The first step when you start running is the start of your exhale, and you count one, two, three, four as you exhale.

Starting on an exhale with a decent volume of air in your lungs before you begin moving means controlling the exhale is easier as you get into the starting rhythm you need for that SBR. There are also times when you might find a 3:3 SBR more comfortable or a 4:4. When you're transitioning between the ratios it's important to allow your breathing to be relaxed and fluid rather than stuck or feeling restricted to a set ratio. Explore and experiment to see what feels right for you.

Anaerobic training session

We've learned how we can use breathing in long easy aerobic runs, and pacing strategies with the SBRs, so now let's look at more anaerobic-based sessions that potentially make up 20% of your training plan or weekly routine: interval sessions, hill reps and sprint sessions.

As anaerobic-based sessions aren't continuous in nature like aerobic sessions, we have a recovery period between the reps of intervals, hill reps or sprints. Ask yourself if you want to maximise recovery during the session or if the purpose of the session is to challenge your recovery to get better at it. We'll look at differences between different sessions and give guidance on how best to use the breathing techniques we've learned.

Interval sessions and recovery

Let's take the popular 4×4 Norwegian method I mentioned earlier, where you run at intervals of four minutes at a high intensity, 85–95% of max heart rate. Typically, this is beyond our ventilatory and lactate thresholds in zone 5, with three minutes of rest between reps.

It's highly likely that nasal breathing in any form is not possible at this intensity. If you're working hard enough, not only will we see heart rate ramp up to 85–95% of your max, even if you are not wearing a watch or heart rate monitor, the intensity is likely be at the point you have to mouth breathe. At these higher intensities and faster-paced sessions, using a hybrid of active exhales from Ian Jackson's Breathplay with the high 2:2 SBR can be really effective. It's great for regulating your speed of breathing and enhancing running economy because, remember, you get some 'free work' of the diaphragm from those ground reaction forces when your breathing and foot strike are in sync. Finally, it's particularly effective for managing the larger quantities of carbon dioxide that you'll be generating at those higher work intensities.

In the three-minute recovery between the four reps of four-minute efforts, your job is to try and get your heart rate back down. The quicker you can get your heart rate down, the better your recovery will be between reps and the harder you'll be able to go in the next rep. So, in this scenario we are going to optimise recovery and choose to make it as easy as possible, as the focus on the session is on hitting that high-intensity effort during each four-minute rep. It's not a session designed to make recovery harder to create an adaptation – as it would have a negative effect on the next rep, and although it might feel harder, it won't be a truly high-paced effort because you won't have recovered sufficiently.

The three-minute rest period is a great opportunity to use the IRBP (intra-recovery breathing protocol) from chapter 12.

Key points to remember:

- Initially dump carbon dioxide to help you get better control of your breathing rate and tidal volume.
- Use your mouth initially, as breathing will be hard, but gradually revert to nasal breathing.
- When nasal breathing again, gradually gain control of the speed of your breathing and use deeper diaphragmatic breaths to help slow the rate down.
- Finally, start to gradually extend your exhalations when it feels comfortable to do so. Don't force it too much or you'll make yourself feel out of breath – find the Goldilocks in your exhales.

The first time I did this session at the end of my final four-minute effort, when I was absolutely exhausted, my heart rate was 180bpm, which is apparently beyond max for a 42-year-old (at the time), so, yeah,

I was working hard! After one minute, where I initially dumped carbon dioxide and used my mouth to get control of my overall breathing rate, my heart rate was down to 150bpm, then after two minutes, I'd got back to nasal breathing and could slow the exhales a little, and my heart rate was down to just 120bpm. It had come down 60bpm from max at 180bpm to just 120bpm in two minutes, which is well within zone 1 for my heart rate. I felt so much better so quickly. I felt in control.

As I did, with this protocol you should see that within the three-minute recovery, you gain control of your breathing faster, feel less out of breath and, importantly, lower your heart rate faster than if you allowed your breathing to stay on auto. Remember that your auto setting doesn't want you to recover well so you can go and smash another interval, no. The auto setting wants you to stop and get on the sofa. And that's not what strong runners do!

Nasal threshold intervals

This is a different type of interval specifically for improving your threshold of nasal breathing. From the final assessment in chapter 7, you will have determined the pace you can manage nasal breathing, the tipping point before you have to open your mouth – your NT. That switch point is trainable and changeable. As you integrate all the breathing techniques into your training, you'll see that naturally improve. You can also do some specific intervals to give your NT a real boost!

The key parameter for these types of intervals is that you're working at between 80% and 90% of your nasal threshold pace. This feels challenging but you can stay relaxed because it's just under your threshold.

- Calculate 80–90% of your NT pace.
- Start with 30-second reps at that pace, followed by a 30-second recovery jog.
- Perform five reps of two sets with a two-minute active recovery between sets – keep it nasal!

You can gradually build up to reps of one minute of 80–90% of your NT with a one-minute recovery jog. Eventually you can even integrate it into traditional interval sessions that are in your training programme, as long as the efforts are below your NT. Or you can use a few reps of these as a nice warm-up for harder intervals, where you might gradually use your mouth more as you ramp the intensity up.

Sprint sessions or hill sprints

Repeated-sprint sessions and hill sprints are a great way to build anaerobic conditioning, improve lactate threshold and VO_2 max. The purpose of the session is to create a strong anaerobic stimulus. Very simply, the stronger the stimulus, the stronger the adaptation. If we can expose ourselves to less oxygen and more lactate in those types of sessions – yes, be warned, they will feel harder – we'll create some stronger adaptations.

How do you reduce oxygen and increase lactate in a sprint or hill session? Remember the 'Czech locomotive', Emil Zátopek, who held his breath during training? Yep, as French scientist Xavier Woorons showed, just four weeks of repeat-sprint training with exhale breath-holds resulted in an improvement in repeat-sprint ability by a factor of 10. Repeat-sprint training with exhale breath-holds leads to increased lactate and decreased muscle oxygenation, resulting in improved clearance and tolerance of lactate and enhanced reoxygenation in recovery periods.[7]

How do you do it?

Firstly, it's important that you do it safely. Avoid this type of training if you have any cardiovascular illness, disease, high blood pressure or if you're pregnant. Start easy and make the breath-holds progressive, building up gradually, and only do one or two sessions at most per week.

There are two ways I programme breath-holds into athletes' conditioning programmes: where the sprint is dictated by the breath-hold, or where the breath-hold is integrated into the start of the sprint.

Type 1: Breath-hold dictates the sprint

In this type of session, you set a sprint distance (like Woorons did in his 2018 study) of around 40m and you try to hold your breath for the entirety of the sprint. The breath-holds are on an exhalation, not an inhalation, and around 40m might take somewhere between six and seven seconds, or faster depending on your speed, which is manageable for most fit and healthy runners without any prior practice.

The challenge comes in the rest periods. I always make the breath-holding progressive, in other words, start with longer rest intervals and gradually reduce them over time. A typical example would be starting with an exhale breath-hold sprint every 60 seconds. So, if the sprint lasts six seconds to cover 40m, then you get 54 seconds of rest. A typical starting point would be two sets of four or five repetitions with three minutes of active recovery between sets.

As you adapt and improve, you can gradually reduce the interval times from every minute to every 45 seconds, where if your sprint lasted seven seconds, you'd get 38 seconds of recovery, reducing the intervals down to every 30 seconds. The less time for recovery, the harder the next exhale breath-hold sprint becomes.

Type 2: Integrated breath-holds

In this type of session, you simply integrate the exhale breath-hold into the start of the sprint you are performing in your session.

For example, I have a hill outside my house that I like to use as hill sprint training, which takes about 45 seconds to run up. There is no way I can run all of it holding my breath. But what works well is starting each repetition with an exhale breath-hold and holding as long as I can, taking my breath-hold to break point. When you get to the point where you can't hold your breath any longer, breathe, but continue to finish – in this case, the hill sprint. It provides a really strong stimulus of increased lactate that you feel almost immediately in your legs, but your body adapts over time, and you get better.

There is an added bonus in this type of session that you don't have to change your existing sprint, interval or hill session – you simply integrate this into the start of each rep. Something I love to emphasise is when you let go of that breath-hold mid-rep, you want to gasp for air, you want to pant, your breathing rate wants to go crazy. Your breathing mechanics want to jump into your chest (rather than utilising your diaphragm), but you can choose how you respond. You know it's coming. It's not a surprise and you can choose how you breathe. Stay calm and practise maintaining focus under stress when out of breath. It's a great opportunity to practise controlling your breathing with good mechanics when your natural inclination is telling you otherwise.

These types of high-intensity sprint or hill anaerobic-type sessions are tough. The intensity is high, so treat them with the respect they deserve. Ensure if you are providing the extra stimulus, you are doing the extra recovery and down-regulation work to respect it – see down-regulation practice from chapter 12.

You can even use breath-holds as part of your warm-up if you are feeling a bit 'flat' ahead of a session. Studies have shown the exhale breath-holds to effectively increase sympathetic activity of the nervous system due to their up-regulating nature providing a spike in heart rate and energy.[8] They are especially helpful, I find, before afternoon sessions when we might feel typically more lethargic.

Race or event day

Have you done your homework?
Marc Swinbank had the goal of running the milestone sub-3-hour marathon, and we developed a programme integrating the different breathing techniques into his various training runs throughout his weekly schedule. He did his homework and reaped the benefits at the Barcelona marathon.

'Breathing was a game changer in my journey to running a sub-3-hour marathon in Barcelona,' he said. 'Learning how to slow my breath, stay calm under pressure, and breathe from my diaphragm in a much more controlled and efficient way was key.' But it wasn't always the case that Marc found controlling his breathing easy despite being a very accomplished amateur runner. 'Before working on my breathing, I'd often end up gasping for air way too early in my runs. Jacko helped me switch to a smoother, more natural way of breathing that's made a huge difference – not just in training, but on race day too. I managed to finish in 2:57, feeling strong and steady right to the end. Honestly, I never thought something as simple as breathing could have such a big impact, but it really has!'

One of the key things – before we go into the differences between 5–10km events and marathons and half marathons, and ultra-marathons – is understanding the difference between using breathing to make adaptations, as we've discussed, compared to using breathing to optimise your performance in a race or event.

You have a few tricks up your sleeve, such as CO_2 dumps and the power of your diaphragm, for when you are in a race. You can even do things like quieten your breathing to psychologically mess with your opponents. Like elite fell runner Ellis Bland described, making them worry that you're not even finding the pace difficult. When you hear them starting to pant, that's when you put the afterburners on.

The most important factor remains staying relaxed, and we know how breathing can directly impact that in everything from your warm-up to when you are pushing your limits and feel out of breath. Race day is about calming nerves by managing your nervous system and dialling in focus to execute your race. It is not a time for training your breathing – it is about using your breathing to maximise your performance.

If you've been doing your homework, you've hopefully truly changed your auto. In that case, whether you're nasal or mouth breathing, you'll still be using your diaphragm, mechanically ventilating efficiently, sufficiently oxygenating your muscles and, importantly, you'll be in control of your breathing rate. You're more efficient, just like the elites. When you're more efficient, you save energy, you're more economical and you're more relaxed.

When you've done the homework, you've changed the auto. You can relax. Just breathe. Just run.

Now, that said, there are some distinct differences between different distance events and races where you'll benefit from being aware of appropriate ways to use your breathing to optimise your success in that type of event.

Calming pre-race nerves and de-stressing

Before we jump into which breathing strategies to adopt in races of varying distances, we're going to look at how we can use breathing to regulate our nervous system to calm pre-race nerves. I want to help you get into a calm, relaxed, de-stressed state ready for optimal performance and entering flow state.

A pioneer in the sporting world for regulating the nervous system is Dr Sally Needham, a human development, performance and culture consultant. She uses contemplative neuroscience to help athletes understand their natural stress response, the resulting behaviours and how to control their nervous system to their advantage. She explained, 'Breathing is one of the biggest tools that we've used to help athletes regulate, which can be simple things like extending exhales. A player making their premier league football debut used breathing to help manage nerves and stay regulated and reflected that without the breathing techniques we'd taught them, they wouldn't have been able to process the experience.'

Anna Harding from The Running Channel explained to me she uses the same Garmin that helps track her runs to help her with things like calming pre-race nerves, as well as getting off to sleep and even de-stressing in airports. She uses the Breathwork widget on her Garmin watch, which has a variety of breathing exercises and guides you when to inhale and exhale. She successfully used it to calm her nerves ahead of the Amsterdam marathon when she was gunning for a new marathon PB, breaking the four-hour barrier coming home in 3:52 – a new PB.

When we calm our breathing, we calm our nervous system and mind. As England Rugby player Bevan Rodd experienced, despite initially being sceptical when we started working together. He explained, 'I never really believed in breathing exercises. They always seemed like a waste of time – too simple to make any real difference. But after trying them during a stressful period, everything changed. Just a few minutes each day brought unexpected calm and clarity. My mind slowed down, my heart stopped racing, and I felt more in control. It's amazing how something so basic can have such a deep impact. Breathing with awareness has helped me manage anxiety, sleep better, and stay grounded. I'm genuinely surprised by the difference it's made. I wish I'd started sooner, it's truly opened my eyes.'

The breath is a simple and a powerful tool, but it certainly isn't complicated. You might have an app or a watch like Anna Harding, with a breathwork option that uses speed to help guide calming breathing, but you don't need the expensive technology. There are some simple steps you can easily take which are key to this:

- **Focus on nasal breathing** – nasal breathing helps slow and calm our breathing naturally and improves focus and concentration.
- **Quieten the breath** – when we breathe quietly, we naturally breathe slower, which regulates the nervous system and calms any pre-race nerves.
- **Depth of breath** – once breathing is calm and slow, focus on feeling the depth of breath with the movement of your diaphragm drawing air into the lower portion of the lungs (just remember: deep doesn't mean big).
- **Slow the exhale** –once the breath is calm, quiet and deep, start to gradually slow down the exhales to extend them and access the relaxation response.

In the race

5–10km – faster running

In a shorter-distance race such as 5–10km, you'll more than likely be working at an intensity beyond your 80–85% VO_2 max and, therefore, potentially beyond your NT. The more homework you do to improve your NT, the more you'll see that switch point increase.

However, don't feel like you have to keep it nasal if you feel restricted, as long as you've done your homework and earned the right to mouth breathe.

At that point, remember:

- Work your mouth like a nose and ensure that you are still mechanically ventilating efficiently.

- Use your diaphragm to increase tidal volume.
- Keep control of your breathing rate.

As you push your own new limits, with Math Roberts ringing through your ears, 'this is how it's meant to feel', you can relax knowing, yes, when you are pushing yourself, it's going to feel hard, but you don't have to panic or stress out – you can relax knowing that you are breathing hard but efficiently, and it's meant to feel like this.

To help maintain that all-important relaxation, we have two tricks in our arsenal when we are starting to push our limits in these faster-paced shorter-distance races.

- Using a medium (3:4) or high (2:2) SBR can help you maintain a rhythm, reduce work of the diaphragm, stay focused and in flow state.
- Unleashing active exhales can be helpful if the build-up of carbon dioxide is making you feel breathless.
- You can then combine the higher SBRs with active exhales for your final push to the finish line, helping you maintain form and gain that extra burst of speed in a sprint finish towards your new PB!

Half and marathon – longer running

During longer distances you might find that a greater proportion of your run is done breathing nasally, depending on your switching point and the nature of the terrain or event route. Regardless of whether you are using your nose or mouth, as always, using your diaphragm and controlling your breathing rate are key to breathing efficiency and staying relaxed. In these types of distances, as you are pushing your limits for a much longer period of time than in a 5km or 10km race, staying relaxed as you become increasingly fatigued can be difficult. Using breathing to both pace yourself and find a rhythm can be a game changer for staying relaxed and feeling less out of breath.

The low or medium SBRs can be extremely effective in the early stages of the race before switching to the high ratio towards the latter part of the race (if you need it) as you make your final push. The LRC that SBRs are based on help manage pacing, reduce perception of fatigue and find a meditation-like rhythm and flow. It's been transformative for many, magical almost – a gateway into flow state, which helps with that all-important relaxation.

Let's look at these two key aspects for longer races: pacing and flow state.

- **Pacing** – In the early part of longer-distance races, if you are prone to going off too fast or struggle with pacing in general, using low or medium SBRs will help you manage your pacing and energy levels early on in the race, especially if you can manage it nasally.
- **Flow state** – Getting into flow state is key not just to an impressive performance but also to an enjoyable race. Managing as much of the early part of the race (or all of it if you like/can) nasally helps with achieving a flow state.

Something that can knock us out of flow state is a disruption to our rhythm, be that in our stride or breathing. Many runners have reported losing rhythm and relaxation when they feel more out of breath after taking a gel or a drink during a longer-distance race, such as a marathon. One undeniable benefit of nasal breathing during running means that you can breathe and drink without disruption to your rhythm.

It doesn't mean you have to do your entire run breathing nasally, but if you can improve nasal breathing when running, you won't feel like you have to gasp for air after taking a drink, and it will help you maintain rhythm and relaxation.

Ultra-marathons – stupidly long running

The ability to self-regulate is one of the fundamentals to ultra-marathons where breathing really comes into its own. That means regulating your pace as well as your nervous system. And especially if it's a multi-day event – the better you can regulate your nervous system, the better you can recover, the better you sleep, and the better chance you have of actually being able to perform the next day. Instead of finding yourself crying in the toilets with your pants round your ankles calling for your mummy. Yes, that happened to me at the start of my final day in my first multi-day ultra!

Using your breathing to stay regulated with your pace so you don't burn out too early is a skill ultra-runner and Peloton coach Susie Chan is familiar with. She explains, 'I use my breathing to know how I'm feeling. It indicates how fatigued I am, rather than changes in heart rate. Using breathing as an indicator of RPE, can I talk, am I in control? It's a simple and free way to regulate effort.' Susie Chan started running ultras back in 2010 before they were 'cool'. She's run the Marathon Des Sables four times and spoke of the need to 'save as much energy as possible' on ultras, especially on these multi-day events. During events in hot climates like Marathon Des Sables, 'you lose a lot of moisture through your breath', and when you're running through a desert, dehydration and cramps can be a big problem. One thing about nasal breathing is that it helps retain more moisture than mouth breathing, so you can use it as a hack to stay better hydrated during long hot events.

Keys to staying regulated during the race

- Regulate the speed and control of your breathing.
- Use nasal breathing to regulate the stress response when possible.
- During any downhill or easy part of the route, get back to nasal breathing and start to calm your breathing to lower heart rate and aid recovery.

It's not only a game changer in these stupidly long ultras, but it's also essential if you want to take on a challenge that pushes you well outside your comfort zone. The reason many of us take on ultra-marathons is because we want to push our physical abilities beyond what we've previously experienced and believed possible.

Everyone says it, and those of us that have done ultra-marathons know the mind is ultimately the thing that will make or break the event. If you can't self-regulate the nervous system, the mind will start to play tricks on you. But when you can self-regulate, the mind becomes your biggest weapon.

I experienced this during my first UTMB World Series Event in 2025 – a 100km race (which, unnecessarily, covered 106km) with over 6500m of elevation across tricky mountain terrain.

It was personally my best performance to date in an ultra-marathon of this magnitude. Worryingly, I'd earned the right to mix it with the big boys, which meant I was in the first wave setting off at 4:30 a.m. with the elites in the field, which included Mathieu Blanchard, who flew up the first of eight mountains on the route.

My aim was to not just finish this brutal ultra, but I wanted to complete it in a respectable time. I needed to regulate my nervous system as much as possible.

I deployed everything possible with my breathing to manage what turned out to be 19 hours 55 minutes of physical torture, but it was an event that I enjoyed psychologically more than any other race to date. Regulating my nervous system with my breathing not only helped me physically perform far beyond anything I'd ever done before but also enjoy it all at the same time.

At every opportunity I tried to:

- Manage pacing and energy with nasal breathing and a low SBR during flatter sections and medium SBR during runnable climbing sections.
- Regulate 95% of the climbs with nasal breathing.
- Use carbon dioxide dumps on the toughest climbs to regulate the speed of my breathing.
- Get back to nasal at the top of the climbs.
- Regulate my breathing rate on the descents to lower heart rate and aid recovery.
- Use nasal breathing, which helped me stay focused and in rhythm even when taking on important electrolyte drinks and eating fuel throughout the race. During a 100km race like this you need to drink and eat a lot of fuel. If you can't nasal breathe when running, you can't easily eat and drink when on the move because you have to nasal breathe when eating and drinking!

I came in as the 99th male, five minutes under my target time of 20 hours, and I couldn't have been happier or prouder of my physical and mental performance – by far, my greatest running achievement to date.

Not bad for a 43-year-old ex-rugby player, recovering from a traumatic brain injury.

Experiences in running such as this continue to cultivate my belief that we are far more capable than we allow ourselves to believe. When we are able to self-regulate, think clearly, stay focused and limit the stress response, we open up new avenues of potential that have always been inside us. It's our breathing that's the first domino in releasing us from that restrictive stress response.

I know this because I've also experienced the other side of it. Letting the stress response take over your breathing and take over your mind. You end up hating the experience, wishing your way to the finish line, wasting energy on hating yourself and the choices you made (especially the one where you signed up to the race in the first place).

Multi-day ultras: Nervous system regulation

It's not just regulation of your pace in multi-day ultra-endurance events. It's also about regulating your nervous system to manage the stress of hours and hours of running, because it can be very hard to allow the body to switch off and sleep if you are too 'up-regulated' from the day's running. 'I tried the down-regulation you taught us but my body couldn't switch off,' explained Ollie Marchon after the Trans Alpine Trail over seven brutal days in the Alps.

The same thing happened to me during my first multi-day ultra, before I was experienced. Down-regulation to help with recovery and sleep doesn't start once the day's running has finished, and no matter how much humming you do, your nervous system is so fired up it won't allow you to switch off. When your stress from training or an event outweighs your recovery, you're going to be in a bad place, which can either make or break a multi-day ultra-event or a hard block of training. Crying on the toilet at my sister's house at the start of day three on the Ring O' Fire (a three-day, 213km ultra-marathon) was a sign I'd not regulated well. I tried my down-regulation at the end of days one and two, but I just couldn't do it. My body and mind were so stressed, the down-regulation humming didn't even touch the sides.

We need to be regulating during the run itself. It takes a bit of practice, and we all have our limits, but with training we are all capable of more. My most recent challenge in 2025 pushed me to new limits: I ran two marathons a day up the entire west coastal path of Wales from St David's Head in the south to Caernarfon castle in the north. Staying regulated through the six-day challenge was essential: monitoring my pace and nervous system with low and medium SBRs was vital during the day when running two marathons up 13,000m of elevation (across the week). Better regulation of my nervous system during the day while running two marathons allowed me to actually down-regulate at night to help improve what little sleep I was able to get.

Integrating into your training

Now, getting better is about integrating some of these techniques into your current training. Practice is key. It's necessary to change the auto. Practice requires you to think about your breathing while running, but, long term, when you change the auto, you don't have to think about it in the race. When you've practised in training, it happens more naturally in a race or event. If you've done enough homework, you'll have changed your auto, so it just happens, and you just run.

Start by identifying which types of training sessions you think you could use to practise some of the techniques. What is the focus of the session? Is it aerobic or anaerobic? Do you want to make recovery easy or challenge it? Then select the appropriate technique and start integrating it into those sessions.

We said we'd look at the difference between integrating breathing practice into different training sessions and applying the techniques in different races. You've learned some principles to apply to your training, as well as two simple questions to ask yourself about the session you're about to embark on when choosing the appropriate breathing technique to optimise your adaptations.

Whether you are looking to take part in your first 5km, set a PB for a half marathon or take on a seemingly impossible ultra-event, I hope you feel equipped to integrate breathing smarter into your training to transform yourself into a stronger runner.

Key takeaways

- Strategies during training runs versus race day may differ when you are trying to create an adaptation by integrating an appropriate breathing technique.
- Understanding the purpose of a training run allows you to use the appropriate breathing technique during both the run itself and in recovery periods. Choose the right breathing tool for the adaptation that you're aiming to achieve in that session.
- On race day, relaxation is key, and this starts before the running begins. Calming your breathing pre-race helps calm the nervous system and any nerves.
- Depending on the distance of the race, different strategies can be used to optimise breathing and oxygen efficiency as well as relaxation. Just make sure you've done your homework by practising them through integration into your training.

> Jacko's breathwork helped me defend my world title, because I was always in control of the effort, I was in control of my body and in total control of my mind. It meant I could relax, enjoy and express myself on the world stage.
>
> **Sam Ruddock, double World Champion Paralympic Cycling**

CHAPTER 14

The golden rules

Breathing within training has been long overlooked due to a lack of research and misconceptions within science about its influence. Yet the tide is turning and the money we've been leaving on the table is within everyone's grasp. Pieces of the breathing puzzle are falling into place. We're forming a picture of calm, controlled, well-regulated breathing, resulting in a more efficient, resilient, stronger runner.

What if we throw the kitchen sink at it?

You never go back to the scene of the crime. I've never been back to the Sheffield parkrun where I set the PB that ignited this journey. Part of me wants to keep it that way, but another part of me wants to go back and see what adaptations I've made since then. The PB I ran was one minute three seconds faster, and I'd only been working on some basics of nasal breathing and controlling the rate of my breathing, trying to increase my tidal volume for four weeks. A bit like the study with the runner who trained nasally for six weeks and improved their 5km time trial by 6%.[1] Six per cent off a 20-minute 5km is about 1 minute 14 seconds. That's a crazy amount of time to drop off a 5km PB. I did similar in four weeks and I'd only just started.

I didn't even know what I was doing back then. My ribcage was still all jacked up, as I'd not come across any of the breathing mobilisations discussed in chapter 9. I had no clue what a diaphragm contraction felt like. I'd not discovered the energy-saving and hypnotic rhythmic nature of LRC to relax me into flow state. It's been over six years since that parkrun in Sheffield. Maybe I should go back armed with my new auto setting, increased carbon dioxide tolerance, improved running form – thanks to a better ribcage position, a stronger diaphragm, a more mobile ribcage – and looser hip flexors and breathing hacks, such as turtle power and carbon dioxide dumps, to allow me to really throw the kitchen sink at it! It intrigues me to know what the compounding effect of stacking all the breathing techniques together would have on a comparative run. A bit like a great team, where the sum of the parts is greater than the individual components, I feel the same is true when you put all the pieces of our breathing puzzle together.

Maybe I will go back one day.

The biggest piece of the puzzle

When trying to be smarter at breathing to improve running, it's critical we control our breathing rate rather than letting our breathing control us.

Breathing smarter to become a stronger runner is about being smart with the way we improve the control of our breathing rate. To be able to regulate the speed, we have, in fact, very few options to choose from. Slowing down an ever-increasing breathing rate during running really comes down to being able to do what we see with elite runners – breathing deeper with the diaphragm and a larger tidal volume. To do that, we must be able to control the urge to breathe, which increases the faster or longer we run.

Training to reduce our urge to breathe requires us to down-regulate chemoreceptors to carbon dioxide through tolerance training, as well as activating the mechanoreceptors in the lungs and ribcage with a stronger, better positioned diaphragm and mobilised ribcage.

Our other option is to become more efficient with our breathing and running economy so we don't actually need to breathe as much to achieve the same oxygenation, as we can extract more oxygen per breath when we ventilate more efficiently. This in itself requires us to be able to control our breathing rate, as a slightly slower, yet slightly deeper and larger breathing cycle improves alveoli ventilation and ventilation efficiency.

Not only that, we can actually be more efficient, so we need less oxygen and air to do the same amount of work. In that instance (having created adaptations from training our breathing), we simply don't need to breathe as hard because we don't need as much air. Breathing is calm and relaxed. Our mind is calm and our body relaxed.

We combine all three when we breathe smarter while becoming stronger runners. The key is integrating it into your training so you create those adaptations.

Making changes is about making it stick

It can be easier to integrate the appropriate breathing strategy into various types of training runs and events than you might think, especially when you start to feel the benefits and your automatic habits begin to change. This is one of the keys to 'making it stick'. To make changes to your breathing to transform your running, we need to make it consistently easy to integrate. That's my job as a coach.

It's not a case of 'oh, not another thing I have to think about', which is how some runners have initially responded before they've understood, appreciated and felt the benefits of breathing smarter. It's not another thing to do – you are already breathing, obviously, on any and every run you go on. Are you in control of your breathing or is your breathing in control of you? It's either working for you or working against you.

If we aren't intentional, it's natural and easy to allow the stress response to restrict our breathing. Equally, with some practice, we can take advantage of using breath control to optimise and improve your performances both in training and events or races.

Yes, in the initial stages you will need to place more awareness on your breathing than you have before, but that's not a bad thing. For example, the rhythmic flow of LRC, synchronising breaths with steps, is going to help you relax and guide you effortlessly into flow state as you lose track of time. Using a tool like LRC is going to feel better, make running easier and you'll want to do it more. Even better, once you've done enough of your homework and truly changed your auto setting, you won't have to think about it at all. It will happen naturally and effortlessly, just like it does for the elites.

Like anything, we need to practise to get the best out of it. When it's easy to do, it becomes part of your training rather than a chore that you have to make time for. Once consistent with practice, you start to feel the benefits, and then you want to keep integrating it regularly into various running sessions. That's what makes it stick.

When it sticks, it changes the auto.

What have we learned from the science?

Wasn't it interesting to learn researchers have recently performed a U-turn on the belief that the lung is overbuilt for exercise, despite Professor Dempsey highlighting this back in 1985? It's interesting to note what science has missed over the years, particularly for us runners. The lung is potentially only just about able to cope with intensities up to 85% of VO_2 max, which, either by design or coincidence, is the same value that most noses can manage in an exercise test.

It's been a breath of fresh air seeing more recent research acknowledging and exploring the effects of various types of breathing strategies on exercise performance. We are now starting to take that knowledge to make informed decisions about which of the holes in our face to use and in what circumstances.

Science has also studied elites and the way they breathe during running compared with untrained or amateur runners. The differences that we've seen lay the foundations for the recipe we can use to breathe smarter like the elites, and maybe one day run a bit more like them too!

What have we learned from elites?

Physiological and psychological differences

Elite athletes appear to have a lower ventilatory response to hypercapnia (high carbon dioxide), meaning they tolerate carbon dioxide better during running and know how it's meant to feel. Overall, their breathing rate is more controlled, giving them a reduced perception of effort and better relaxation.

What research can't answer is whether elites are naturally gifted with high carbon dioxide tolerance or if it's a training adaptation. I know where my inclination lies, and the reality might be that it's a bit of both. Whether it's a cause or correlation for the elites, we know increasing our carbon dioxide tolerance helps reduce our urge to breathe during running, which allows us to control our all-important breathing rate. It not only impacts our physiology but also our psychology, and we've got the breathing protocols to integrate into our training sessions to improve it.

How they ventilate – not *how much*

The key to elite runners' efficient breathing is the way they ventilate, rather than just ventilating more air. Their increased tidal volume, combined with the stretch of the mechanoreceptors in the diaphragm, lung wall and ribcage, helps reduce air hunger sensations, resulting in a slower breathing rate and reduction in perception of effort and improved relaxation.

The larger tidal volume and controlled breathing rate creates a deeper breath that enables more air to reach the alveoli sacs low down in the lungs, creating a more efficient breathing cycle, with more oxygen extracted with each breath. Elite runners increase their tidal volume, through controlled breathing, all the way to exhaustion, while amateurs are restricted by their tidal volume, meaning they have to breathe faster and faster.

If our ribs are tight and our diaphragm restricted, we are fighting a losing battle when trying to increase our tidal volume in the same way as an elite. I'm not even qualified to tie the shoelaces of an elite runner, but through mobilising my ribcage, I've started to benefit from increasing my tidal volume all the way to exhaustion. For example, during my VO_2 max test my tidal volume rose from 1.95 litres at the start gradually and continually all the way to 2.91 litres and 2.92 litres in the final two 30-second increments of the test. We need to start using the breathing mobilisation to allow our ribcage to expand, which will also help unleash our superhero: the diaphragm.

The diaphragm is their superpower

When using the power of the diaphragm, elite runners pull air down into the lower lobes of the lungs where there's a greater density of alveoli, which takes longer and allows for a greater diffusion of oxygen from the lungs into the blood. Essentially, when we breathe more like an elite runner, we extract more oxygen per breath, so we don't have to do it as much or as hard because we improve ventilatory efficiency. As we don't require as much air, our respiratory rate reduces, reducing sympathetic nervous system activity and potentially cardiovascular stress. We can also relax more, perceive less effort, reduce fatigue and feel more in control.

We've also seen the important role diaphragmatic breathing plays in improved posture, running form and force transfer. When the ribcage is positioned correctly, with pressure in the 'canister' rather than bracing our core, we start becoming stronger runners. It can even reduce tension in the stomach, release tight hips and melt away pain in some cases.

Synchronisation of running and breathing

Synchronising the beautiful rhythm of their breathing with the relaxed effortless rhythm of their running is something elite runners appear to do naturally. The identified benefits of LRC are appetising in theory and mind-blowing in practice.

When the foot strike is synchronised with the contraction of the diaphragm, the downward pull from ground reaction forces assists the diaphragm, as it contracts downward on an inhale. This reduces the effort for the thousands of times the diaphragm contracts on a run, which reduces respiratory muscle fatigue, especially on longer or more intense runs. In theory this sounds great, and with practice, feels amazing when you get it right. Part of that amazing feeling is being drawn into a hypnotic trance, hearing your foot kissing the floor as you listen to the sound of your breath. You're in flow state without realising it. You have no idea how long it's been or how you got there. You're beyond that all-important relaxation. You're lost in the moment!

Easy means easy

When around 80% of our training is supposed to be done in zone 2, it should be easy, but everyone out there wants to go fast like Ricky Bobby from the film *Talladega Nights*. Not the elite runners. On their easy runs, they are running easy. The pace should be comfortably below your NT. Remember what Michael Crawley observed with Ethiopia's finest runners, in *Out of Thin Air*: 'so serene at this pace, he's breathing through his nose'.[2]

When we're doing zone 2 runs, we can keep the pace relaxed by choosing to use the nose. Breathing through the nose during this pace is not only natural, better for your heart and a more efficient form of breathing, but it also helps guide pacing. If you are in tune with the subtle feedback your breath gives you about oxygenation and lactate – which have an inverse relationship – you can control your heart rate zone with pinpoint accuracy.

All of the pieces of our puzzle: Techniques, protocols and hacks

Ultimately, relaxation is the key domino to improving our running, and our breathing is an essential piece of the relaxation puzzle and the gateway to flow state. But breathing is far more than just a tool to use for relaxation in a run.

All the breathing techniques we've learned can be split into categories: breathing before running, during races, during training for adaptation or breathing for recovery after running.

To learn how to benefit from breathing like the elites, you need to do your homework by training breathing to create adaptations in the appropriate training sessions. The assessments in chapter 7 should have given you a good idea of which areas are most important for you.

It is important to appreciate that all the techniques elite runners use are all things we can train. Let's break down the different tools we can deploy:

Calm your nervous system with calm breathing. We can use our breathing to prepare and start our run in a calm and de-stressed state. Of all the things to improve, relaxation has always been top of our list. Our ability to stay relaxed when running starts with being able to de-stress from the baggage of daily life. Focusing on calm, quiet nasal breathing for just a few minutes can transform our state so that before we start running, we are calm, relaxed and ready to enter flow state.

Train your airway by training your tongue. Our tongue is a hidden gem, the link between our airway and diaphragm that can not only improve the function of our airway but also the superhero of inhalation, our diaphragm. Unfortunately (until now) the tongue has been overlooked as a muscle that affects breathing. When we train our tongue, we reduce restriction of the airway, strengthen its structural integrity, and improve our capacity for nasal breathing. The tongue is also connected to the diaphragm, through the deep front line of fascia, helping improve breathing mechanics when positioned correctly in the roof of the mouth. This improves your breathing during running, at rest and, importantly, during sleep when your airway relaxes along with all our muscles. Calmer breathing at night creates a calmer nervous system as you sleep. Better sleep equals better recovery.

Unlock and train your diaphragm. The diaphragm is the key muscle of inhalation, but its power goes beyond improving just our ventilation efficiency by drawing air into the lower portions of the lungs. Stronger and more optimal functioning of the diaphragm not only allows for an increase in tidal volume, it also provides vital stability in our core, which helps transfer ground reaction forces and improves running economy. When your diaphragm is stronger, you're a stronger breather and become a stronger runner.

Mobilise your ribcage to improve your capacity to breathe and move. The mobility of your ribs affects the mobility of your spine, which affects the position of your ribcage and your posture. This can either optimise your running form or restrict it, along with your breathing capacity. Our thoracic spine plays a key role in maintaining a tall running posture, and as our ribs connect to it, there is a direct relationship between breathing and the spine. The position of the diaphragm is dictated by the ribcage, which houses it. As the diaphragm is connected through fascia to key muscles around the hips, the breathing mobilisation exercises can transform your respiratory capacity and hip mobility, even reducing pain in the tightest of runners' hip flexors. Better mobilisation of the ribs also allows you to increase tidal volume, help control breathing rate, and reduce perception of effort and breathlessness by stretching mechanoreceptors in the lungs and ribcage.

Synchronise breathing and running to improve running economy and access flow state. Using LRC might just be the simplest tool that will transform more than one component of your running. The hypnotic nature of the simple task, syncing your foot strikes with your breath cycle, provides little dopamine hits each time you get the reward of your left and right foot strike swapping on each exhale, which provides all the ingredients to achieve flow state. The timing of the inhales with your foot strike allows for what scientists describe as 'free energy', by using ground reaction forces to reduce the load on the diaphragm. This helps reduce respiratory muscle fatigue, which is especially important for longer runs or races.

Breath-holds to improve carbon dioxide and lactate tolerance. Holding your breath after an exhale during running isn't going to make that specific anaerobic session, hill sprint or interval any easier, but it will create training adaptations not only to your lactate tolerance but also lactate clearance and reoxygenation during recovery periods. The carbon dioxide you're not letting out of your lungs over time will improve your tolerance to it, giving you greater capacity to control your all-important breathing rate.

Regulate your nervous system for improved recovery. Conscious control of our breathing can help reduce heart rate for improved recovery both during (IRBP) and after (PRBP) training sessions or runs. When we control our exhales, we can reduce our heart rate during recovery periods in harder training session faster and more effectively. For post-run recovery and to help improve sleep (or between days on multi-day ultras), we can use breathing to regulate our nervous system to enhance recovery with down-regulation humming.

Plus, you'll still have a few tricks up your sleeve and some hacks, such as CO_2 dumps and turtle power, for an extra boost whenever you need it.

Stacking techniques

Each breathing technique, like a single piece of paper, doesn't hold much weight on its own, but as Aristotle is believed to have said, 'The whole is greater than the sum of its parts.' Stacking breathing techniques together unleashes an unstoppable force within you.

Layering the basics of good tongue posture helps with our airway as well as postural stability.[3] The position of our ribcage also helps with running form, as well as torquing up the fascia, which not only helps with effortless propulsion but also connects your diaphragm with your tongue for more efficient diaphragmatic breathing.

When we add the synchronising of our steps and breath, not only does it mean a reduced workload for the diaphragm – which delays fatigue and any potential blood stealing (metaboreflex) – we are combining free energy from the fascia system for our propulsion with free energy for our diaphragm. Runners report back that both running and breathing both feel easier.

Stacking breathing techniques is like putting more pieces of our puzzle together. The more pieces of the puzzle we have in place, the clearer the picture becomes. When the right techniques are stacked together for your particular run, you help improve your running economy. It takes less effort to run fast and ultimately improves how relaxed you look and feel. You look more like an elite and you start to feel like one.

The antisocial (nasal) running club

One of the hot topics of discussion we've covered is which hole in your face to breathe through. Too often the conversation on breathing is overly simplified as to whether you should use your nose or your mouth. We've seen from the extensive list of breathing techniques that better breathing goes way beyond just a choice between which hole in your face to use.

That said, this is such an important aspect, and because it impacts many other components, such as the speed and depth of our breathing, it deserves its own little section. Having clarity on the 'nose v mouth' debate is key to appreciating it's never a black or white answer. Making the right choice depends on you individually and the purpose of your run.

Benefits of nasal breathing

One of the great benefits of nasal breathing is the calming effect it has on slowing your breathing before you start your run. Beginning your run in a calmer state makes it easier to start with a sense of that all-important relaxation, so picking your nose (not literally) – meaning closing your mouth and breathing through your nose before you start running – is a no-brainer when it comes to preparing for your run.

Dr Martin Yelling spoke of using calming slow breathing exercises in his coaching to help reduce the stress that daily life challenges all levels of runner he's worked with over the years. Ellis Bland described using breathing exercises to calm pre-race nerves and Paralympic champion Richard Whitehead spoke of using breathing to 'dial in' and focus during warm-ups. Using nasal breathing pre-run and in your warm-ups is great for calming your stress levels and preparing the mind for what's ahead.

Using nasal breathing to help pace easy sessions is one of the most frequently used benefits. The pace that someone can nasal breathe appears to have some correlation with their heart rate zone 2. Rather than constantly looking at your watch, you can listen to your breathing, which doesn't disrupt your rhythm and can even guide you into flow state more easily. Trying to keep it nasal and allowing your nose to dictate the pace of your next easy run or zone 2 session might be the best yet simplest thing you can do. If you find it hard initially, remember you have some tricks up your sleeve, like turtle power, which can increase total nasal ventilation by 26%. It might also be useful to have a tissue up your sleeve initially, as the nose can be especially runny when you first start using it more.

The biggest mistake people make with nasal breathing is sucking air up the nose and making it stressful. Firstly, remember the nasal cavity canals go backwards and not up, and when you breathe up your nose, you hike up the ribcage inefficiently. Put your tongue up and breathe back. Secondly, your nose isn't a hoover, so don't use it like one! The resistance the nose provides is a great tool for strengthening your diaphragm, but not to the point that it becomes stressful and you can't ventilate enough air.

Health benefits

Picking your nose over your mouth and joining the nasal running club has some very important health benefits, particularly for those enjoying running for the purpose of improving their health.

Nasal breathing may help protect the heart in endurance runners, who are potentially more susceptible to scarring of the heart tissue, according to Professor Dallam and respiratory scientist Martin McPhilimey. The reduction of stress and slow breathing rate with nasal breathing also has a de-stressing effect on your body and mind in general. The function of the nose and the nitric oxide it produces also helps protect your airways and lungs, which if you suffer from asthma, can be life-changing, as I've seen with many clients. You also reduce your likelihood of becoming ill with respiratory infections, allowing you to be more consistent with training.

The antisocial side of nasal breathing!

The only downside of nasal breathing is it requires you to keep your mouth shut, which is a little antisocial if you're in a group or with a friend, as you can't talk! It's been well documented that using a conversational pace is a good way to regulate your pace to stay in zone 2, which I'm not disagreeing with. However, when you're talking, you're mouth breathing, and that's less efficient for your conversational-paced zone 2 runs, so it's somewhat counterproductive.

I saw the direct effect of this on a run with my mate Harvey. I'd not seen him for ages and was excited to tell him all about the nasal breathing I'd been practising as we set off on a 10km easy run. The irony was, as I excitedly spoke about nasal breathing being more efficient, I was doing a lot of talking and therefore a lot of mouth breathing! The end result was for the same pace I'd usually run a 10km my heart rate was 10bpm higher. All the talking was mouth breathing which led to a faster breathing and heart rate. Although, sometimes in life talking to your mate is far more important than the efficiency of your breathing.

For those who like the meditative state of running alone, you'll find using nasal breathing on those easy runs will help you access flow state and feel present as you listen to the hypnotic sounds of your breath and foot strike. When out with friends on easy runs, you either become the best listener anyone has ever run with or run the risk of being considered antisocial as you are not talking.

Earn the right to mouth breathe

Earning the right to mouth breathe really is the cornerstone of my philosophy. Rather than allowing mouth breathing to be an automatic compensation – essentially your brain trying to get you to stop – we can use our knowledge to make better use of the bigger hole in our face. To do that you need to practise controlling your breathing rate so you can access your diaphragm. The resistance from your nose can actually be helpful in training your diaphragm and that important breath control.

Your nasal breathing is the training ground. It's the workout for your respiratory system as a whole, whereas the mouth is an easy option. Easy options don't lead to strength, growth and progress. That said, beyond your NT, the mouth comes into its own. It allows you to ventilate larger volumes of air per breath and, if you've done our homework, you'll still be doing it efficiently rather than as a compensation. It feels like you've got an extra gear or a turbo boost when you open your mouth and reduce the restriction from the nose while maintaining all the elements of efficient breathing that keep you regulated and relaxed.

Like the subject in the 2019 study who, after six weeks of nasal-only training, when allowed to use the extra gear (his mouth), dropped his 5km time from 17:27 to an astonishing 16:22. Just like my story in the introduction, he knocked off over a minute of his 5km time.[4] It's exciting to think what you might achieve yourself!

Excitingly, as I continue to explore the benefits hidden in our breath, we've started planning a study with Dr Robins and researchers at Salford University using the techniques that we've outlined to show the effects not just on my VO_2 max data but on a range of runners. It's part of my commitment to get better at understanding the relationship between breathing and performance as we embark on our quests to become stronger runners. Together, we will move forward, and the more we explore, the more we'll uncover – I'm sure of it. History has taught us that.

If we have to boil it all down to the most important ingredients in our puzzle of using breathing to transform our running, with relaxation as the holy grail, what would they be?

The biggest domino that influences everything, from the efficiency of your breathing, your mental state, perception of effort and regulation of your nervous system, is your breathing rate. Are you in control of your breathing or is your breathing controlling you?

There are three key pillars I've identified that underpin everything you are trying to achieve. In order of importance, these are:

- Breathing rate
- Diaphragmatic breathing mechanics
- The holes in your face

I've pointed out throughout this book there's clearly been things with breathing we've overlooked in the past. It would be ignorant of me to not think I'm doing exactly the same now. History has always shown us that we are always slightly wrong. We used to think the world was flat, it sort of is in places, but it's not the full picture. I'm sure there's more pieces of the breathing puzzle we'll discover but hopefully the picture is at least a little clearer.

My encouragement is to be like Professor Dempsey, who challenged the current way of thinking that the lung was overbuilt for exercise in the 1980s. Question everything, experiment with the practical application outlined in this book. Test it. Play with it. See how it changes your breathing, your performance, or if it changes anything at all. Even when it doesn't make it better, that is still progress because finding out something doesn't work for you isn't failure, it's progress to finding out what does, because you're one step closer. It might even simply be that you need more practice at it before you'll notice the differences.

Finally then, a question from me for you. What will you do with your new smarter breathing? Does becoming a strong runner mean a new PB in your 5km, maybe your first half or even full marathon, or could you push yourself to test your body and mind over an ultra-marathon?

I'd love to hear from you. Please share your experiences with the breathing techniques integrated into your training and the effects it has on your running and what challenges you're taking on! Email any stories or questions to jacko@thebreathrunningcoach.com or connect with me on Instagram @thebreathrunningcoach.

It's a bit of a secret as I write this, but my next challenge will be a world record attempt running 200 marathons in 100 days, throughout Great Britain, starting summer 2026. I will be using all of the techniques outlined in this book for what we are calling 'Mission IN-possible', in order to run two marathons every day for 100 days. I *need* to use all of these breathing tools to have a chance to redefine my impossible.

When you regulate your body and mind with your breath, you'll change the impossible to IN-possible. What possibilities might open up to you, when your breath shifts your mindset?

> Engaging in breathwork sessions with Jacko brought a transformative shift in my approach to running. Rather than pursuing performance metrics as end goals, I began to see running as a practice to refine my breathing and enhance biomechanical efficiency. By learning how to consciously influence my oxygenation and regulate my mental state through breath, I unlocked new levels of physical potential – especially in foot power, diaphragmatic strength, and ribcage alignment.
>
> These changes translated into a more grounded, efficient and resilient running form, allowing my body to move with greater ease and endurance. This integration of breath awareness not only improved my running form but also had a positive ripple effect on both my overall health and professional clarity.
>
> **Sarah Mohr, runner, artist and coach**

Breathe Smarter, Run Stronger checklist

Here's a summary of our breathing techniques for your run. Take a photo or screenshot so you can refer back to it before or during your warm-up.

Whether you breathe through your nose or mouth, synchronise your steps with your breath, or dump carbon dioxide or not, the breathing tools you select depend on your distance and speed, your current progress and the purpose of the session. But these three points remain in place as pieces of our puzzle to breathing smarter:

1. **Control your breathing rate** – helps regulate your mind, relax your body and breathe more efficiently.
2. **Ribcage stacked on top of the pelvis** – optimises your diaphragm and running posture.
3. **Inhalation driven by the diaphragm** – enhances efficiency of breathing, stability in your canister and improves force transfer.

Pre-run – Calm, quiet nasal breathing with slower exhales to calm the nervous system and de-stress.

Warm-up – Breathing mobilisation to free up your ribcage and activate your diaphragm.

Start of run – Keep breathing nasally to start with to help guide pace, dial in your focus, warm up your diaphragm and access flow state. Remember:

- Tongue up.
- Breathe back (not up the nose like a hoover!).

During run
- Turtle power – increase nasal ventilation by 26%.
- LRC – SBRs: 4:5, 3:4 or 2:2.
- Active exhales with the mouth when intensity ramps up.
- Carbon dioxide dumps – to help you get back to nasal during recovery.

References

My story
1. Froman C. 'Alterations of Respiratory Function in Patients With Severe Head Injuries'. *British Journal of Anaesthesia* (1968), 40, 354.

Chapter 1
1. Nicolò A, Massaroni C, Passfield L. 'Respiratory Frequency During Exercise: The Neglected Physiological Measure'. *Frontiers in Physiology* (2017), 8, 922.
2. 'Your Lungs and Exercise'. *Breathe* (Sheff) (2016), (1), 97–100.
3. Romano C, Nicolò A, Innocenti L, Bravi M, Miccinilli S, Sterzi S, Sacchetti M, Schena E, Massaroni C. 'Respiratory Rate Estimation during Walking and Running Using Breathing Sounds Recorded with a Microphone'. *Biosensors* (2023), 13, 637.

Chapter 2
1. Harms C, Wetter T, St Croix C, Pegelow D, Dempsey J. 'Effects of Respiratory Muscle Work on Exercise Performance'. *Journal of Applied Physiology* (1985), 2000, 89, (1), 131–138.
2. Harbour E, Stöggl T, Schwameder H, Finkenzeller T. 'Breath Tools: A Synthesis of Evidence-Based Breathing Strategies to Enhance Human Running'. *Frontiers in Physiology* (2022), 13, 813243.
3. Migliaccio G, Russo L, Maric M, Padulo J. 'Sports Performance and Breathing Rate: What Is the Connection? A Narrative Review on Breathing Strategies'. *Sports (Basel)* (2023), 11, (5), 103.
4. Benzie, S. *The Lost Art of Running*. (Bloomsbury Sport, 2020), 209–210.
5. Shimozawa Y, Kurihara T, Kusagawa Y, Hori M, Numasawa S, Sugiyama T, Tanaka T, Suga T, Terada RS, Isaka T, Terada M. 'Point Prevalence of the Biomechanical Dimension of Dysfunctional Breathing Patterns Among Competitive Athletes'. *Journal of Strength and Conditioning Research* (2023), 37, (2), 270–276.
6. Harbour E, Stöggl T, Schwameder H, Finkenzeller T. 'Breath Tools: A Synthesis of Evidence-Based Breathing Strategies to Enhance Human Running'. *Frontiers in Physiology* (2022), 13, 813243.
7. Shimozawa Y, Kurihara T, Kusagawa Y, Hori M, Numasawa S, Sugiyama T, Tanaka T, Suga T, Terada RS, Isaka T, Terada M. 'Point Prevalence of the Biomechanical Dimension of Dysfunctional Breathing Patterns Among Competitive Athletes'. *Journal of Strength and Conditioning Research* (2023), 37, (2), 270–276.

Chapter 3
1. Nicolò A, Gruet M, Sacchetti M. 'Editorial: Breathing in Sport and Exercise: Physiology, Pathophysiology and Applications'. *Frontiers in Physiology* (2023), 14, 1347806.
2. Blackie S, Fairbarn M, McElvaney N, Wilcox P, Morrison N, Pardy R. 'Normal values and ranges for ventilation and breathing pattern at maximal exercise'. *Chest* (1991), 100, (1), 136–42.
3. Lucía A, Carvajal A, Calderón F, Alfonso A, Chicharro J. 'Breathing pattern in highly competitive cyclists during incremental exercise'. *European Journal of Applied Physiology and Occupational Physiology* (1999), 79, 512–521.
4. Blackie S, Fairbarn M, McElvaney N, Wilcox P, Morrison N, Pardy R. 'Normal values and ranges for ventilation and breathing pattern at maximal exercise'. *Chest* (1991), 100, (1), 136–42.
5. Gravier G, Delliaux S, Delpierre S, Guieu R, Jammes Y. 'Inter-Individual Differences in Breathing Pattern at High Levels of Incremental Cycling Exercise in Healthy Subjects'. *Respiratory Physiology & Neurobiology* (2013), 189, (1), 59–66.
6. Lucía A, Carvajal A, Calderón F, Alfonso A, Chicharro J. 'Breathing pattern in highly competitive cyclists during incremental exercise'. *European Journal of Applied Physiology and Occupational Physiology* (1999), 79, 512–521.
7. Rovelli, C. *There are places in the world where rules are less important than kindness*. (Allen Lane, Penguin Books, 2020), 68.
8. Carli M, Peters J, Dempsey, Susan, Hopkins A, Sheel W. 'Is the Lung Built for Exercise? Advances and Unresolved Questions'. *Medicine & Science in Sports & Exercise* (2023), 55, (12), 2143–2159.
9. Harbour E, Stöggl T, Schwameder H, Finkenzeller T. 'Breath Tools: A Synthesis of Evidence-Based Breathing Strategies to Enhance Human Running'. *Frontiers in Physiology* (2022), 13, 813243.

10. Ibid.
11. Ibid.
12. West J. *West's Respiratory Physiology: The Essentials*. 11th Edition. (Wolters Kluwer, 2021), 143.
13. Bassett J, Howley E. 'Maximal Oxygen Uptake: "Classical" Versus "Contemporary" Viewpoints'. *Medicine & Science in Sports & Exercise* (1997), 29, (5), 591–603.
14. Costill DL, Thomason H, Roberts E. *'Fractional utilization of the aerobic capacity during distance running'*. Med Sci Sports. 1973 Winter;5(4):248–52. PMID: 4774203.
15. Bassett D Jr, Howley E. 'Limiting Factors for Maximum Oxygen Uptake and Determinants of Endurance Performance'. *Medicine & Science in Sports & Exercise* (2000), 32, (1), 70–84.

Chapter 4

1. Papp L, Klein D, Gorman J. 'Carbon Dioxide Hypersensitivity, Hyperventilation, and Panic Disorder'. *American Journal of Psychiatry* (1993), 150, (8), 1149–1157.
2. Malhotra V, Hulke S, Bharshankar R, Chouhan S, Ravi N, Patrick K. 'Effect of Slow and Deep Breathing on Brain Waves in Regular Yoga Practitioners'. *Mymensingh Medical Journal* (2021), 30, (4), 1163–1167.
3. Clarke D, Sokoloff L. 'Regulation of Cerebral Metabolic Rate'. In: Siegel G, Agranoff B, Albers R, Fisher S, Uhler M, (editors). *Basic Neurochemistry: Molecular, Cellular and Medical Aspects*. 6th Edition. (Lippincott-Raven, 1999).
4. Convertino V, Ryan K, Rickards C, Glorsky S, Idris A, Yannopoulos D, Metzger A, Lurie K. 'Optimizing the Respiratory Pump: Harnessing Inspiratory Resistance to Treat Systemic Hypotension'. *Respiratory Care* (2011), 56, (6), 846–857.
5. Harbour E, Stöggl T, Schwameder H, Finkenzeller T. 'Breath Tools: A Synthesis of Evidence-Based Breathing Strategies to Enhance Human Running'. *Frontiers in Physiology* (2022), 13, 813243.
6. Woorons, X. *Hypoventilation Training*. (ARPEH, 2014).
7. Berner R, 'Atmospheric Oxygen Over Phanerozoic Time'. *Proceedings of the National Academy of Sciences* (1999), 96, (20), 10955–10957.
8. Pleil J, Ariel Geer Wallace M, Davis M, Matty C. 'The Physics of Human Breathing: Flow, Timing, Volume, and Pressure Parameters for Normal, On-Demand, and Ventilator Respiration'. *Journal of Breath Research* (2021), 15, (4), 10.1088/1752-7163/ac2589.
9. Ibid.
10. Ibid.
11. Harbour E, Stöggl T, Schwameder H, Finkenzeller T. 'Breath Tools: A Synthesis of Evidence-Based Breathing Strategies to Enhance Human Running'. *Frontiers in Physiology* (2022), 13, 813243.
12. Woorons, X. *Hypoventilation Training*. (ARPEH, 2014).
13. Brinkman J, Toro F, Sharma S. 'Physiology, Respiratory Drive'. [Updated 2023 Jun 5]. In: *StatPearls* [Internet]. (StatPearls Publishing, Jan 2025). Available at: https://www.ncbi.nlm.nih.gov/books/NBK482414/
14, 15 and 16. Ibid.
17. Campbell E. 'The Effect of Muscular Paralysis Induced by Curarization on Breath Holding in Normal Subjects'. *American Review of Respiratory Disease* (1979), 119, (2P2), 67.
18. Kayser B, Sliwinski P, Yan S, Tobiasz M, Macklem P. 'Respiratory Effort Sensation During Exercise With Induced Expiratory-Flow Limitation in Healthy Humans'. *Journal of Applied Physiology* (1997), 83, (3), 936–947.
19. Marcora S. 'Perception of Effort During Exercise is Independent of Afferent Feedback From Skeletal Muscles, Heart, and Lungs'. *Journal of Applied Physiology* (2009), 206, (6), 2060–2062.
20. Supinski G, Clary S, Bark H, Kelsen S. 'Effect of Inspiratory Muscle Fatigue on Perception of Effort During Loaded Breathing'. *Journal of Applied Physiology* (1987), 62, (1), 300–307.
21. Lansing R, Im B, Thwing J, Legedza A, Banzett R. 'The Perception of Respiratory Work and Effort Can Be Independent of the Perception of Air Hunger'. *American Journal of Respiratory and Critical Care Medicine*. (2000), 162, (5), 1690–1696.
22. Nicolò A, Massaroni C, Passfield L. 'Respiratory Frequency During Exercise: The Neglected Physiological Measure'. *Frontiers in Physiology* (2017), 8, 922.
23. Salazar-Martínez E, de Matos T, Arrans P, Santalla A, Orellana J. 'Ventilatory Efficiency Response is Unaffected by Fitness Level, Ergometer Type, Age or Body Mass Index in Male Athletes'. *Biology of Sport* (2018), 35, (4), 393–398.
24. Dallam G, McClaran S, Cox D, Foust C. 'Effect of Nasal Versus Oral Breathing on VO_2 max and Physiological Economy in Recreational Runners Following an Extended Period Spent Using Nasally Restricted Breathing'. *International Journal of Kinesiology and Sports Science* (2018), 6, 22.
25. Pleil J, Ariel Geer Wallace M, Davis M, Matty C. 'The Physics of Human Breathing: Flow, Timing, Volume, and Pressure Parameters for Normal, On-Demand, and Ventilator Respiration'. *Journal of Breath Research* (2021), 15, (4), 10.1088/1752-7163/ac2589.

26. Ibid.
27. Sun X-G, Hansen J, Garatachea N, Storer T, Wasserman K. 'Ventilatory Efficiency during Exercise in Healthy Subjects'. *American Journal of Respiratory and Critical Care Medicine* (2022), 166, (11), 1443–1448.
28. Harbour E, Stöggl T, Schwameder H, Finkenzeller T. 'Breath Tools: A Synthesis of Evidence-Based Breathing Strategies to Enhance Human Running'. *Frontiers in Physiology* (2022), 13, 813243.
29. Bossé Y, Côté A. 'Asthma: An Untoward Consequence of Endurance Sports?'. *American Journal of Respiratory Cell and Molecular Biology* (2020), 63, (1), 7–8.
30. Seltmann C, Killen L, Green J, O'Neal E, Swain J, Frisbie C. 'Effects of 3 Weeks Yogic Breathing Practice on Ventilation and Running Economy'. *International Journal of Exercise Science* (2020), 13, (2), 62–74.
31. Clifton C, Killen L, Green J, O'Neal E, Swain J, Frisbie C. 'Effects of 3 Weeks Yogic Breathing Techniques on Sub-maximal Running Responses'. *International Journal of Exercise Science* (2023), 16, (4), 1066–1076.
32. Murphey J, Lafrenz A, 'Effects of Nasal Only and Apnea Breathing on Performance in Trained Cyclists'. *International Journal of Exercise Science: Conference Proceedings* (2020), 8, (8), Article 5.

Chapter 5

1. Harbour E, Stöggl T, Schwameder H, Finkenzeller T. 'Breath Tools: A Synthesis of Evidence-Based Breathing Strategies to Enhance Human Running'. *Frontiers in Physiology* (2022), 13, 813243.
2. Ibid.
3. Dallam G, Kies B. 'The Effect of Nasal Breathing Versus Oral and Oronasal Breathing During Exercise: A Review'. *Journal of Sports Research* (2020), 7.
4. Dallam G. *The Nasal Breathing Paradox During Exercise*. (Innovative Ink Publishing, 2024).
5. Dallam G, Kies B. 'The Effect of Nasal Breathing Versus Oral and Oronasal Breathing During Exercise: A Review'. *Journal of Sports Research* (2020), 7.
6. Thomas S, Phillips V, Mock C, Lock M, Cox G, Baxter J. 'The Effects of Nasal Breathing on Exercise Tolerance'. *Chartered Society of Physiotherapy Annual Congress* (2009), Oct 16, 2009.
7. LaComb C, Tandy R, Ping Lee S, Young J, Navalta J. 'Oral Versus Nasal Breathing During Moderate to High Intensity Submaximal Aerobic Exercise.' *International Journal of Kinesiology and Sports Science* (2017), 5, 8–16.
8. Niinimaa V, Cole P, Mintz S, Shephard R. 'The Switching Point From Nasal to Oronasal Breathing'. *Respiration Physiology* (1980), 42, (1), 61–71.
9. Dallam G, Kies B. 'The Effect of Nasal Breathing Versus Oral and Oronasal Breathing During Exercise: A Review'. *Journal of Sports Research* (2020), 7.
10. Dallam G. *The Nasal Breathing Paradox During Exercise*. (Innovative Ink Publishing, 2024).
11. Allen K, Moris JM, Curtis R, Chang CJ, Arnold B, Koh Y. 'Enhancing Oxygen Uptake Efficiency Through Nasal Breathing in Aerobic Exercise,' *International Journal of Exercise Science*: Conference Proceedings (2024): Vol. 2: Iss. 16, Article 107.
12. Flanell M. 'The Athlete's Secret Ingredient: The Power of Nasal Breathing'. *EC Pulmonology and Respiratory Medicine* (2019), 471–475.
13. Retty T. 'The Effects of Nose-Breathing-Only Training on Physiological Parameters Related to Running Performance: A Case Study'. *BPHE, Nipissing University*, 2019.

Chapter 6

1. Schmidt J, Carlson C, Usery A, Quevedo A. 'Effects of Tongue Position on Mandibular Muscle Activity and Heart Rate Function'. *Oral Surgery, Oral Medicine, Oral Pathology, Oral Radiology, and Endodontology* (2009), 108, (6), 881–888.
2. di Vico R, Ardigò L, Salernitano G, Chamari K, Padulo J. 'The Acute Effect of the Tongue Position in the Mouth on Knee Isokinetic Test Performance: A Highly Surprising Pilot Study'. *Muscles Ligaments Tendons Journal* (2014), 3, (4), 318–323.

Chapter 7

1. Hill A, Kelly E, Horswill M, Watson MO. 'The Effects of Awareness and Count Duration on Adult Respiratory Rate Measurements: An Experimental Study'. *Journal of Clinical Nursing* (2018), 27, 546–554.
2. Martin B, Sparks K, Zwillich C, Weil J. 'Low Exercise Ventilation in Endurance Athletes'. *Medicine and Science in Sports* (1979), 11, (2), 181–185.
3. Kowalski, T et al. 'Body Oxygen Level Test (BOLT) is not associated with exercise performance in highly-trained individuals'. *Frontiers in Physiology* (2024), Volume 15.

4. Garner M, Attwood A, Baldwin DS, James A, Munafò MR. 'Inhalation of 7.5% Carbon Dioxide Increases Threat Processing in Humans'. *Neuropsychopharmacology* (2011), 36, (8), 1557–1562.
5. Shimozawa Y, Kurihara T, Kusagawa Y, Hori M, Numasawa S, Sugiyama T, Tanaka T, Suga T, Terada RS, Isaka T, Terada M. 'Point Prevalence of the Biomechanical Dimension of Dysfunctional Breathing Patterns Among Competitive Athletes'. *Journal of Strength and Conditioning Research* (2023), 37, (2), 270–276.
6. Michaelson J, Brilla L, Suprak D, McLaughlin W, Dahlquist D. 'Effects of Two Different Recovery Postures during High-Intensity Interval Training'. *Translational Journal of the ACSM* (2019), 4, (4), 23–27.
7. St Pierre S, Peirlinck M, Kuhl E. 'Sex Matters: A Comprehensive Comparison of Female and Male Hearts'. *Frontiers in Physiology* (2022), 22, 13:831179.
8. Farha S, Asosingh K, Laskowski D, Hammel J, Dweik RA, Wiedemann HP, Erzurum S. 'Effects of the Menstrual Cycle on Lung Function Variables in Women With Asthma'. *American Journal of Respiratory and Critical Care Medicine* (2009), 180, (4), 304–310.
9. Murphy W. 'The Sex Difference in Haemoglobin Levels in Adults – Mechanisms, Causes, and Consequences'. *Blood Reviews* (2014), 28, (2), 41–47.
10. Schaeffer MR, Mendonca CT, Levangie CM, Andersen RE, Taivassalo T, Jensen D. 'Physiological Mechanisms of Sex Differences in Exertional Dyspnoea: Role of Neural Respiratory Motor Drive'. *Experimental Physiology* (2014), 99, (2), 427–441.
11 and 12. Ibid.
13. Saaresranta T, Polo O. 'Hormones and Breathing'. *Chest* (2002), 122, (6), 2165–2182.
14. Schmalenberger K, Eisenlohr-Moul T, Jarczok M, Eckstein M, Schneider E, Brenner IG, Duffy K, Schweizer S, Kiesner J, Thayer J, Ditzen B. 'Menstrual Cycle Changes in Vagally-Mediated Heart Rate Variability are Associated with Progesterone: Evidence from Two Within-Person Studies'. *Journal of Clinical Medicine* (2020), 9, (3), 617.

Chapter 8

1. Nason L, Walker C, McNeeley M, Burivong W, Fligner C, Godwin J. 'Imaging of the Diaphragm: Anatomy and Function'. *Radiographics* (2012), 32, (2), E51–70.
2. Harbour E, Stöggl T, Schwameder H, Finkenzeller T. 'Breath Tools: A Synthesis of Evidence-Based Breathing Strategies to Enhance Human Running'. *Frontiers in Physiology* (2022), 13, 813243.
3. West J. *West's Respiratory Physiology: The Essentials.* 11th Edition. (Wolters Kluwer, 2021), 117.
4. Ibid.
5. Zwoliński T, Wujtewicz M, Szamotulska J, Sinoracki T, Wąż P, Hansdorfer-Korzon R, Basiński A, Gosselink R. 'Feasibility of Chest Wall and Diaphragm Proprioceptive Neuromuscular Facilitation (PNF) Techniques in Mechanically Ventilated Patients'. *International Journal of Environmental Research and Public Health* (2022), 19, (2), 960.
6. Bhatnagar A, Sharma S. 'Effectiveness of Chest PNF and Breathing Exercises on Pulmonary Function and Chest Expansion in Male Smokers'. *Indian Journal of Physiotherapy and Occupational Therapy - An International Journal* (2021), 16, 159–168.
7. West J. *West's Respiratory Physiology: The Essentials.* 11th Edition. (Wolters Kluwer, 2021), 118.
8. Michaelson J, Brilla L, Suprak D, McLaughlin W, Dahlquist D. 'Effects of Two Different Recovery Postures During High-Intensity Interval Training'. *Translational Journal of the ACSM* (2019), 4, (4), 23–27.
9. Harbour E, Stöggl T, Schwameder H, Finkenzeller T. 'Breath Tools: A Synthesis of Evidence-Based Breathing Strategies to Enhance Human Running'. *Frontiers in Physiology* (2022), 13, 813243.
10. Bahenský P, Malátová R, Bunc V. 'Changed Dynamic Ventilation Parameters as a Result of a Breathing Exercise Intervention Program'. *The Journal of Sports Medicine and Physical Fitness* (2019), 59, (8), 1369–1375.

Chapter 9

1. Hodges P, Heijnen I, Gandevia S. 'Postural Activity of the Diaphragm is Reduced in Humans When Respiratory Demand Increases'. *The Journal of Physiology* (2001), 537 (Pt 3), 999–1008.
2. Kolář P, Sulc J, Kyncl M, Sanda J, Cakrt O, Andel R, Kumagai K, Kobesova A. 'Postural Function of the Diaphragm in Persons With and Without Chronic Low Back Pain'. *Journal of Orthopaedic and Sports Physical Therapy* (2012), 42, (4), 352–362.
3. Bradley H, Esformes J. 'Breathing pattern disorders and functional movement'. *International Journal of Sports Physical Therapy* (2014), 9, (1), 28–39.
4. Harbour E, Stöggl T, Schwameder H, Finkenzeller T. 'Breath Tools: A Synthesis of Evidence-Based Breathing Strategies to Enhance Human Running'. *Frontiers in Physiology* (2022), 13, 813243.
5. Ibid.

6. Daniels J. *Daniels' Running Formula*. (Human Kinetics, 2014).
7. Harbour E, Stöggl T, Schwameder H, Finkenzeller T. 'Breath Tools: A Synthesis of Evidence-Based Breathing Strategies to Enhance Human Running'. *Frontiers in Physiology* (2022), 13, 813243.
8. Daley M, Bramble D, Carrier D. 'Impact Loading and Locomotor-Respiratory Coordination Significantly Influence Breathing Dynamics in Running Humans'. *PLoS One* (2013), 8, (8), e70752.
9. Harbour E, Stöggl T, Schwameder H, Finkenzeller T. 'Breath Tools: A Synthesis of Evidence-Based Breathing Strategies to Enhance Human Running'. *Frontiers in Physiology* (2022), 13, 813243.
10. Daley M, Bramble D, Carrier D. 'Impact Loading and Locomotor-Respiratory Coordination Significantly Influence Breathing Dynamics in Running Humans'. *PLoS One* (2013), 8, (8), e70752.
11. Harbour E, van Rheden V, Schwameder H, Finkenzeller T. 'Step-Adaptive Sound Guidance Enhances Locomotor-Respiratory Coupling in Novice Female Runners: A Proof-of-Concept Study'. *Frontiers in Sports and Active Living* (2023), 5, 1112663.
12. Ibid.
13. Harbour E, Stöggl T, Schwameder H, Finkenzeller T. 'Breath Tools: A Synthesis of Evidence-Based Breathing Strategies to Enhance Human Running'. *Frontiers in Physiology* (2022), 13, 813243.
14. Ross C, Blob R, Carrier D, Daley M, Deban S, Demes B, Gripper J, Iriarte-Diaz J, Kilbourne B, Landberg T, Polk J, Schilling N, Vanhooydonck B. 'The Evolution of Locomotor Rhythmicity in Tetrapods'. *Evolution* (2013), 67, (4), 1209–1217.
15. Adams D, Pozzi F, Willy RW, Carrol A, Zeni J. 'Altering Cadence or Vertical Oscillation During Running: Effects on Running Related Injury Factors'. *International Journal of Sports Physical Therapy* (2018), 13, (4), 633–642.

Chapter 10

1. Woorons, X. *Hypoventilation Training*. (ARPEH, 2014).
2. Wendi W, Dongzhe W, Hao W, Yongjin S, Xiaolin G. 'Effect of Dry Dynamic Apnea on Aerobic Power in Elite Rugby Athletes: A Warm-Up Method'. *Frontiers in Physiology* (2024), 14, 1269656.
3. Fornasier-Santos C, Millet G, Woorons X. 'Repeated-Sprint Training in Hypoxia Induced by Voluntary Hypoventilation Improves Running Repeated-Sprint Ability in Rugby Players'. *European Journal of Sport Science* (2018), 18, (4), 504–512.
4. Woorons X, Faucher C, Dufour S, Brocherie F, Robach P, Connes P, Brugniaux JV, Verges S, Gaston A, Millet G, Dupuy O, Pichon A. 'Hypoventilation Training Including Maximal End-Expiratory Breath Holding Improves the Ability to Repeat High-Intensity Efforts in Elite Judo Athletes'. *Frontiers in Physiology* (2024), 15, 1441696.
5. Wendi W, Dongzhe W, Hao W, Yongjin S, Xiaolin G. 'Effect of Dry Dynamic Apnea on Aerobic Power in Elite Rugby Athletes: A Warm-Up Method'. *Frontiers in Physiology* (2024), 14, 1269656.

Chapter 11

1. Recinto C, Efthemeou T, Boffelli P, Navalta J. 'Effects of Nasal or Oral Breathing on Anaerobic Power Output and Metabolic Responses'. *International Journal of Exercise Science* (2017), 10, (4), 506–514.
2. Jackson I. *The Breathplay Approach to Whole Life Fitness*. (Doubleday, 1986).
3. Wojta D, Flores X, Andres F. 'Effect of "breathplay" on the physiological performance of trained cyclists'. *Medicine & Science in Sports & Exercise* (1987), 19, (2), S85.
4. Ibid.
5. Harbour E, Stöggl T, Schwameder H, Finkenzeller T. 'Breath Tools: A Synthesis of Evidence-Based Breathing Strategies to Enhance Human Running'. *Frontiers in Physiology* (2022), 13, 813243.

Chapter 12

1. Michaelson J, Brilla L, Suprak D, McLaughlin W, Dahlquist D. 'Effects of Two Different Recovery Postures During High-Intensity Interval Training'. *Translational Journal of the ACSM* (2019), 4, (4), 23–27.
2. Ibid.
3. Gourine A, Ackland G. 'Cardiac Vagus and Exercise'. *Physiology (Bethesda)* (2019), 34, (1), 71–80.
4. Crawley M. *Out of Thin Air*. (Bloomsbury Sport, 2021).
5. Simjanovic M, Hooper S, Leveritt M, Kellmann M, Rynne S. 'The Use and Perceived Effectiveness of Recovery Modalities and Monitoring Techniques in Elite Sport'. *Journal of Science and Medicine in Sport* (2009), 12, S22.
6. Gerritsen R, Band G. 'Breath of Life: The Respiratory Vagal Stimulation Model of Contemplative Activity'. *Frontiers in Human Neuroscience* (2018), 12, 397.

Chapter 13

1. Crawley M. *Out of Thin Air*. (Bloomsbury Sport, 2021).
2. Thomas S, Phillips V, Mock C, Lock M, Cox G, Baxter J. 'The Effects of Nasal Breathing on Exercise Tolerance'. *Chartered Society of Physiotherapy Annual Congress* (2009), Oct 16, 2009.
3. Tucker R, Gearhart S. 'How to Train Like Eliud Kipchoge'. *Runner's World* online, Jun 20, 2023. Available at: https://www.runnersworld.com/uk/training/marathon/a42722004/eliud-kipchoge-training/
4. Holloszy J. 'Biochemical Adaptations in muscle. Effects of Exercise on Mitochondrial Oxygen Uptake and Respiratory Enzyme Activity in Skeletal Muscle'. *The Journal of Biological Chemistry* (1967), 242, (9), 2278–2282.
5. Harbour E, Stöggl T, Schwameder H, Finkenzeller T. 'Breath Tools: A Synthesis of Evidence-Based Breathing Strategies to Enhance Human Running'. *Frontiers in Physiology* (2022), 13, 813243.
6. Ibid.
7. Fornasier-Santos C, Millet G, Woorons X. 'Repeated-Sprint Training in Hypoxia Induced by Voluntary Hypoventilation Improves Running Repeated-Sprint Ability in Rugby Players'. *European Journal of Sport Science* (2018), 18, (4), 504–512.
8. Wendi W, Dongzhe W, Hao W, Yongjin S, Xiaolin G. 'Effect of Dry Dynamic Apnea on Aerobic Power in Elite Rugby Athletes: A Warm-Up Method'. *Frontiers in Physiology* (2024), 14, 1269656.

Chapter 14

1. Retty T. 'The Effects of Nose-Breathing-Only Training on Physiological Parameters Related to Running Performance: A Case Study'. BPHE, Nipissing University, 2019.
2. Crawley M. *Out of Thin Air*. (Bloomsbury Sport, 2021).
3. Alghadir A, Zafar H, Iqbal Z. 'Effect of Tongue Position on Postural Stability During Quiet Standing in Healthy Young Males'. *Somatosensory & Motor Research* (2015), 32, (3), 183–136.
4. Retty T. 'The Effects of Nose-Breathing-Only Training on Physiological Parameters Related to Running Performance: A Case Study'. BPHE, Nipissing University, 2019.

Acknowledgements

There has been too much overwhelming support and encouragement from so many people to name all of them. A special mention has to go to my mum and dad, who saw something in me as a 12-year-old struggling with English at school and sent me to extra English lessons on a Saturday morning, which I hated. But, no doubt, I'd never have been able to write this book without that extra work. I'm not sure they thought I'd write a book, but they believed in me when the schooling system around me didn't.

A special thank you to Matt Lowing from Bloomsbury who saw something in my early writing. You believed in me and, importantly, encouraged me to 'write with no fear', which the 12-year-old boy in me finds liberating. Thank you.

To all the athletes I've had the pleasure of working with who trusted me to help them with something as fundamental and important to their mental and physical performance as breathing. I've always learned so much from them and, ultimately, it's where my coaching process has been honed and developed.

To all the coaches that I've ever worked with or who have coached me. I always feel like my coaching style with athletes is an amalgamation of all the amazing coaches who I've had the chance to work with or alongside. Many of you have no idea of the impact you had on me as both a person and a coach. Thank you especially to Jo Brun and Tim Stevenson.

A special mention is for Patrick McKeown (Oxygen Advantage) whose passion for teaching breathing is something I find infectious, who has been so generous with his time and his teaching for me and thousands of other coaches. He kick-started my breathing education and is someone from whom I continue to benefit from his wisdom to this day. From the bottom of my heart, thank you, Patrick.

Finally, but most importantly, my wife, Catherine, who not only supported me in the writing of this book but supported me through the traumatic brain injury that changed both our lives forever. Thank you for believing in me, seeing more in me than I do and bringing out the best in me.

Index

bold indicates an exercise

4x4 training method, Norwegian 230–2, 241–2
80/20 rule 235–6, 263
   80–85% VO$_2$ 49–53, 56, 57, 87, 94, 95, 98, 204, 235, 249, 260

A

abdominal muscles 157, 167–8
aches and pains 165, 166, 167, 168–70
aerobic training runs
   easy runs: the 80-20 rule 235–6
   step-to-breath ratios 236–41
air hunger 72, 83, 86, 88, 89, 91
airway, upper 98–100, 107
   tongue and airway 101–5, 111–12, 162, 264
   training your tongue and airway 104–6
Alexander, Vassos 110–11, 205
alveolar ventilation 74–5, 79, 89, 259
alveoli 27, 64–5, 68, 74–5, 145–6, 259
amygdala 62
anaerobic training sessions
   interval sessions and recovery 241–3
   nasal threshold intervals 243–4
   sprint sessions or hill sprints 244–6
anxiety *see* de-stressing; stress
arterial oxyhaemoglobin desaturation, exercise-induced 51
Arundell, Henry 229
asthma 75–6, 268
Attia, Dr Peter 235
author's story 99, 164–5
   airway Q-tip experiment 106–7
   brain injury and breathing 20–4, 92–3
   foot strike and breathing synchronisation 169–71
   'Mission IN-possible' challenge 272
   movement analysis and running form 185–8, 198–200
   nasal breathing training 97–8, 99, 109–13
   running in Snowdonia 58–61, 202–3
   Sheffield parkrun 13–15, 257–8
   ultra running and recovery 214–16
Avitabile, Ciaran 79–80

B

Bach-y-Rita, Dr Paul 49
Beach, Nigel 36–7, 61
belly breathing 161
Benzie, Shane 50, 185–7, 195–6, 199, 235
Bland, Ellis 42, 55, 247, 267
blood flow/circulation 25, 69
blood pH 68, 70
blood pressure 25, 69, 196
Bohr effect 69
BOLT score, or control pause 119–21
brain function 22–3, 37, 47–8, 49, 62–3, 67, 69–71, 73, 79, 142, 155, 206
breath-holding 39, 68, 76, 78, 79, 119–21, 189–94, 196–8, 200, 201, 244–6, 265
breathing assessments 115–38
   basic
      autonomic baseline assessments 117, 138
      BOLT score, or control pause 119–21
      resting natural respiratory rate 117–18
   biomechanical assessments 121–2
      active, simulated running 124–5
      diaphragm activation test (DAT) 125–6
      Hi-Lo test — seated *vs* supine 122–3
   nasal threshold (NT) assessment 134–5
   ribcage and movement assessments 127, 174
      assessing hip internal and external rotation 132–3
      assessing hips and hamstrings 132
      checking infra-sternal angle 128
      checking your infra-sternal angle 128
      dos and don'ts 128–9
      ribcage assessment 127–8
      thoracic rotation 130–1, 175

'breathing gears' 207
breathing mobilisations 174–80, 182
   back of ribcage: kneeling posterior mobilisation 174–7
   front of ribcage: exhale floor bridge mobilisation 178–9
   side of ribcage: lunge with reach mobilisation 177–8
   thoracic mobilisation – inhale and exhales combined 179–80

C

calm breathing 224–6, 264
   calm breathing = calm nervous system 224
carbon dioxide (CO_2) 25–6, 27, 64–5, 66, 68–9, 70, 71, 86, 88, 147, 148, 155, 186, 197, 208–9, 218, 232
   the CO_2 dump 210–12, 213, 221, 266
   sensitivity to/tolerance of 24, 62, 68, 72, 73, 76, 77–8, 79, 91, 117, 119–20, 137, 258, 261, 265
Carrera, Davide 62–3
Carreras, Santi 30
central chemoreceptors 69, 155
Central Governor Theory 37, 206
Chan, Susie 251–2
chemoreceptors 69, 71, 155, 208, 228, 258
chest cavity (thorax) 27, 65, 121–2, 145
Clarkson, Fran 201
Cobb, Dr 61, 156, 174
core tension 181–2, 186–7
Costill, David 53
Crawley, Michael 223, 235

D

Dallam, Professor George 40, 52, 53, 74, 85–7, 88, 89, 90–1, 94, 134, 268
Daniels, Dr Jack 171, 236
De Oliveria, Luiz 189
de-stressing 223–6, 248, 264
dead space, pulmonary 75
Decker, Marie 189
Dempsey, Professor 49–50, 56, 94, 260
diaphragm 18–19, 27, 39, 42, 47–8, 64, 66, 70, 72, 76, 78, 89, 91, 92–3, 98, 101, 102–3, 113, 121, 124, 127, 128, 130, 131, 140, 148, 165, 217–18, 258, 262, 264
   anatomy and function 140–4, 163
   breathing mobilisations 174–81, 220
   diaphragm activation test (DAT) 125–6, 151, 162
   and ground reaction force 172
   kinetic chain link 164–5
diaphragmatic breathing 123, 140, 141–2, 145–6, 149, 160–1, 205, 258, 262, 271
   belly breathing mistake 161
   exercises
      blocked inhale 151–2
      exhale bridge 156–60
      progression with 'breath control' 155–6
      starting position – why supine? 150–1
      supine diaphragmatic breathing mechanics 152–4
   external and internal sensations 154
   and hip mobility 167, 168
   position of ribcage 148, 156–60
   role of exhalation 146–7, 163
Dickinson, Dr John 38
Doidge, Norman 49
down-regulation 79, 114, 215, 216–17, 222–6, 227, 229

E

Earls, James 46–7, 140
efficiency, breathing 27, 28–30, 33–42, 44, 47–55, 56–7, 63–7, 73–5, 76
   receptor function and breathing 62, 67–73
   relaxation and breathing rate 57, 61–3, 75, 77, 78
   stacking breathing techniques 266–7
   see also mechanics, breathing; diaphragmatic breathing; mouth breathing; nasal breathing; recovery; relaxation; respiratory rate/breathing rate; tidal volume (V_T)
effort/work sensation 72, 73
Elias, Tess 42, 75–6
elite athletes 31–2, 34–5, 42, 45, 48, 51, 52–3, 56, 62–3, 67, 72–3, 169, 223, 235, 260, 261–3
emotions and breathing 72
energy cost of breathing 53
Evans, Lottie 114
exhalation 27, 66, 68, 70, 71, 86, 140, 142, 266
   exhalation bridge exercises 155–60, 209
   exhale breath-holds 196–7
   and foot strike 167, 169–71, 172–3, 210
   humming 224–6
   intra-recovery breathing 217–18, 220
   mouth breathing 208–10

F

fascia 98, 103, 185–6, 187–8, 195–6, 201, 265
fatigue, muscle 68, 72, 172–3
female physiology 136–7
'fight or flight' stress response 28–9, 61, 62, 79
flexion tone 61, 79
flow state 18, 38, 62, 171, 173, 182, 265
foot and heel pain 169–71
foot strike and breathing synchronisation 167, 169–73, 182–3, 184, 210, 262–3
Ford, George 44
Functional Movement Screen scores 165

G

Galpin, Dr Andy 217
ground reaction force 172

H

Haas, Jennyfer 24
Harding, Anna 41, 248
heart 40, 63, 70, 90–1, 196
heart rate 25, 28, 29, 35, 36, 39, 42, 63, 73, 112–13, 135, 137, 141, 196, 205, 222, 226–7, 266
  importance of regulating 216–17
  see also recovery
Hering-Breuer inflation reflex 70
Hi-Lo test 122–3
Hickson, Kerry 111
hip mobility 131–4, 165, 166, 167, 168–9, 181–2, 184, 265
  assessing hip internal and external rotation 132–3
  assessing hips and hamstrings 132
  see also **breathing mobilisations**
Hoff, Dr Jan 230
hormones, female 136–7
Hughes, Des 75
humming exhales 224–6
hydrogen ions 67, 68
Hypoxia-inducible-factor-1α (HIF-1α) 67
hypoxic/hypoventilation training 189–94, 196–8, 200

I

infra-sternal angle 128
inhalation 26–7, 54, 64, 65, 66, 70, 71, 139–40, 142, 145, 167, 172, 220
intra-recovery breathing 217–18, 220–1, 266
intrathoracic pressure 51

J

Jackson, Catherine 136–7
Jackson, Ian 208–9, 242
Jefferson, Gemma 121, 131, 141, 160, 167–8, 181, 187
Journal of Sports Research 88–9

K

Kipchoge, Eliud 16, 51, 110–11, 206, 235

L

lactate 67, 68, 73, 86, 232, 265
Locomotor-Respiratory Coupling (LRC) 38, 166–7, 169–71, 182–3, 184, 210, 265
  breathing ease 171–3
  finding flow state 173, 265
Lomas, Dr Sebastian 38, 101–4, 105–6
lungs 26–7, 38, 48, 56, 57, 64–5, 67, 66, 70, 71, 72, 89
  alveoli 27, 64–5, 68, 74–5, 79, 145–6
  nasal breathing and protection 75–6
  receptors 70, 76, 258
lymphatic pump, diaphragm as 141

M

MacKenzie, Brian 36, 207
Manners, Jack 184
Marabella, Brian 107
Marchon, Ollie 221–2
Matthews, Alex 78
McKeown, Patrick 9–12, 39, 82, 91, 119
McPhilimey, Martin 37, 46, 72, 90–1, 268
mechanics, breathing 47–8, 65–6, 70, 73, 75, 76, 77–8, 89, 98, 102, 121–6, 168–9
  see also diaphragmatic breathing; ribcage
mechanoreceptors 69, 70, 71, 72, 73, 76, 79, 146, 162, 220, 239, 258, 265
menstrual cycle 137
metabolic acidosis 68
metaboreflex 64
Miller, Jill 142, 174
minimal effort principal 47–8
minute ventilation (V_E) 66–7
Mohr, Sarah 272
mouth breathing 74, 82–3, 86, 89–90, 103, 203, 213, 269–70
  exhalation 208–10
  high intensity training 204, 209–10
  keeping your mouth small 206–7, 209, 213
muscle afferent nerves 67

muscle oxygenation 51, 75, 78, 86
Myers, Thomas 98, 188

N

nasal breathing 24, 52, 74, 75–6, 77, 79, 81–2, 93–5, 163, 204, 205, 236, 267–70
   adaptations from nasal training breathing 88–91
   antisocial side of 269
   breathing backwards *vs* upwards 107–9, 114
   health benefits 90–1, 268–9
   increasing nasal ventilation with turtle power 109–10, 114
   vs mouth breathing 82–3, 85–8, 89–90, 267
   nasal threshold (NT) assessment 134–5
   nasal threshold intervals 243–4
   nose size 83–4, 99
   nostrils 99, 102, 205
   power of the smile - Vassos and Kipchoge 110–11, 114
   research issues 84–5
   training tips 91–2, 97–8, 109–12, 114
   see also airways, upper
Needham, Dr Sally 248
nervous system 24, 25, 28, 44, 62–3, 266
   autonomic 36–7, 61, 62, 82, 137, 141, 215–16, 217
   down-regulation 215–17, 222–6, 266
   regulation during multi-day ultras 254–5
   sympathetic 61, 62
nitric oxide 76, 86, 268
Noakes, Tim 37

O

out-of-breath, feeling 72–3, 83, 171–2
oxygen (O_2) 25, 26, 53–4, 63, 65, 66, 67–8, 69, 70, 73–4, 89, 90, 95
   running and economy of use 53–4, 185–6, 189–94, 196–8, 200, 258–9

P

Partington, Ollie 227
pelvis and diaphragm relationship 166
peripheral chemoreceptors 70
post-recovery breathing and down-regulation 222–6, 227, 266
   calm breathing = calm nervous system 224–6
postural stabilisation and the diaphragm 140, 148, 150, 165

posture and running form 185–8, 195–6, 198–200, 201
pre-Bötzinger complex 69–70
pre-race nerves, calming 248–9
progesterone 136
Pugh, Michaela 138

R

race/event days 257
   5-10km — faster running 249–50
   calming pre-race nerves 248–9
   doing your homework/practice for 246–7
   half- and marathon —longer running 250–1
   multi-day ultras: nervous system regulation 254–5
   staying regulated in the race 252–4
   ultra-marathons 251–2, 254–5
rate of perceived exertion (RPE) 29, 39, 73, 86, 88
receptor function and breathing 62, 67–73, 79, 88
recovery 24, 39, 42, 63, 79, 114, 192–4, 221–2, 227–9, 266
   breathing recovery 'in sessions' 220–1
   importance of heart rate regulation 216–17
   intra-recovery breathing 217–18, 220–1, 226–7
   post-recovery breathing and down-regulation 222–6
   ribcage and breathing recovery 218–19
relaxation and running 30, 36, 44, 57, 61–3, 72, 75, 78, 171, 173, 182, 186–8, 199
respiratory acidosis 68
respiratory rate (RR)/breathing rate 15, 29, 35, 36, 47, 48, 54–5, 61, 65, 66–7, 69, 71, 73, 74, 75, 77, 78, 79, 88, 89, 138, 173, 258, 271
   resting natural respiratory rate assessment 117–18
   see also efficiency, breathing; tidal volume (V_T)
respiratory system
   80-85% VO_2 49–53, 56, 57, 87, 94, 95, 98, 204, 235, 249, 260
   breathing control mechanisms 67–73
   function and physiology overview 25–30, 64–7
   minimal effort principle 47–8
   see also efficiency, breathing; respiratory rate (RR)/breathing rate; VO_2 max

ribcage   47–8, 66, 70, 73, 76, 78, 93, 121, 123–4, 209, 258, 265
   back of ribcage: kneeling posterior mobilisation exercise   174–7
   'chest up and ribs back' cues   195–6
   effect on breathing recovery   218–20
   front of ribcage: exhale floor bridge mobilisation   178–9
   position/alignment   148–9, 156–60, 163, 195–6, 201, 217–20
   relationship with diaphragm   143–4, 145–9, 164–5, 219
   ribcage and movement assessments   127–31
   side of ribcage: lunge with reach mobilisation   177–8
Roberts, Math   59–60, 72, 119, 120, 203
Robins, Dr Anna   68, 87, 270
Rodd, Bevan   248
Rovelli, Carlo   49
Ruddock, Sam   256
Rudisha, David   16, 31–2, 52–3
Runner's World   235–6

S

SAID principle   232–4
Santas, Dana   156, 157, 174
simulated running biomechanical assessment   124–5
Singh Sandhu, Navdeep   175
smiling and nasal breathing   110–11, 114
speed of breathing *see* respiratory rate (RR)/breathing rate
sprint sessions or hill sprints   244
   Type 1: breath-hold dictates the sprint   244–5
   Type 2: integrated breath-holds 245–6
stability, physical   29, 123, 124, 140, 148, 150, 165–7, 168–9, 181–2, 183, 184
stacking breathing techniques   266–7
static breathing exercises   77
step-to-breath ratios (SBRs)   236–41
Stewart, Bob   165–6, 213
stress   25, 28–9, 30, 36–7, 61–2, 78, 114, 166
stride length   167, 168
suction and stretch exercise, tongue and airway   105–6
Swinbank, Marc   163, 246–7

T

Thomas, Iwan   17, 174, 220
thoracic mobilisation   179–80
thoracic rotation movement assessment   130–1, 175
Thorley, Ollie   57
tidal volume (V_T) of breath   47–8, 57, 61, 66–7, 71, 72, 72, 75, 78, 79, 89, 148, 154, 172, 173, 258, 264
tongue   98–9, 101–4, 114, 162, 264
   training your tongue and upper airway   104–6
tracheal dead volume   75

U

ultra running   214–16, 251–2, 254–5

V

vagus nerve   70, 127, 141, 222–3
ventilation   25, 51, 52, 64, 66–7, 69–70
   mechanical   47–8, 65, 75, 76, 77–8, 163
   ventilatory efficiency   52, 64, 73–5, 85–6, 89–90, 95, 259
   ventilatory threshold   87–8
   see also diaphragmatic breathing; efficiency, breathing; nasal breathing; respiratory rate (RR)/breathing rate; volume tidal (V_T)
VHL training *see* hypoxic/hypoventilation training
VO_2 max   204, 235
   levels and breathing efficiency   49–53, 56, 57, 87, 94
   tests   47, 48, 50–1, 52, 74, 83, 87, 89, 109
   ventilatory efficiency test   52

W

warm-ups   77, 79, 184, 234–5
   see also **breathing mobilisations**
West, John   145
Whitehead, Richard   19, 36, 115, 119
Woorons, Xavier   39, 68, 189, 191–4, 197, 220

Y

Yelling, Dr Martin   33, 61, 63, 95, 199, 223, 267

Z

Zátopek, Emil   45, 189
'zone of apposition' (ZOA), diaphragm   145, 148, 154, 163

Praise for *BREATHE SMARTER, RUN STRONGER*

'Learning to breathe better is a game changer for your running.'
Richard Whitehead MBE, Paralympic champion and world record holder

'As a coach and researcher, I am always looking for new ideas and ways to further my understanding. Breathing is foundational to efficient, resilient running, yet few athletes truly understand it. This excellent and informative book fills that gap. It's simple, smart and grounded in real running.'
Shane Benzie, author of *The Lost Art of Running*

'A fascinating read ... simple, exciting insights that will make you run faster and feel more relaxed whilst doing so.'
Paul Tonkinson, author of *26.2 Miles to Happiness*

'Since working with Jacko the impact he's had on my mental and physical feeling has been transformational. The techniques and education he has taught me have opened my eyes into how to breathe properly in certain positions and situations to improve my performance. Whether that's mobility, controlling my breathing in the heat of the game or down regulation breathing, the impact has been absolutely brilliant.'
George Ford, England Rugby player

'Jacko's breathwork helped me defend my world title. Because I was always in control of the effort, I was in control of my body and in total control of my mind. It meant I could relax, enjoy and express myself on the world stage.'
Sam Ruddock, double World Champion in para cycling

'I've been running marathons and coaching marathon runners for 40 years and never once has someone like David (an expert in breathing) explained to me and showed me how I can improve my breathing ... David's book has educated me on that! In this book he presents the benefits of breath mastery with simplicity and clarity.'
Dr Martin Yelling, coach, runner and author of *Running in the Midpack*

'A fantastic guide and learning tool.'
Bob Stewart, England Rugby medical lead, men's senior team

'Jacko is a master-breather! Not only is he an accomplished athlete who has conquered breathwork but Jacko breathes life, energy and clarity into the science of running and respiration ... David tells the story of his injury and his

ensuing exploration into the science of breath with humility, grace and humour. He keeps you turning the pages to find your next step on your journey to mastering breath and making your running easier, more graceful, and in tune with your physiology. Every runner, in fact, every breather will benefit from time spent with this book.'
James Earls, author of *Born to Walk*

'A great blend of science, theory and practical advice.'
Gemma Jefferson, Performance Physiotherapist for Olympic and Paralympic athletes

'Most runners train their legs and overlook their breath. Jacko flips that script. Train your breathing and everything changes: build real endurance, move more efficiently, and recover faster. If you exercise, if you run, if you breathe, this book is for you.'
Matteo Pistono, author of *Breathe How You Want to Feel*

'This is more than a book about how we breathe; it's a training masterclass based on thousands of hours of coaching and personal application. Jacko makes something as complex as respiration, and how we train it for optimal efficiency, accessible to every runner.'
Matt Bagwell, Master Breath Training Instructor and ultramarathon runner

'If you want better performance, start with your breath. In *Breathe Smarter Run Stronger*, Jacko gives you a system to assess, train, and apply your breathing in a simple, repeatable way. It improves not only how you run but, more importantly, how to stay composed when running gets hard.'
Carl Paoli, author of *Freestyle Connection*

'A game-changer. Jacko's story from professional rugby player, sustaining a brain injury, to breathwork coach and ultra-runner is simply inspiring. The book also achieves a goal that many authors aspire to, that of explaining a technical subject or science in everyday language, blending science and practice to clearly explain how breathing affects endurance, recovery, and mental focus ... a must-read for runners interested in being a better athlete and also becoming more connected to their body and its performance.'
Matt Ward, Runcomm

'This book is a breath of fresh air for the performance world, offering an updated scientific perspective on how athletes can practically integrate this work into their training.'
Martin McPhilimey, respiratory scientist

Learn more from Jacko at
www.thebreathrunningcoach.com

Follow breath training programmes by Jacko at
www.probreathwork.com

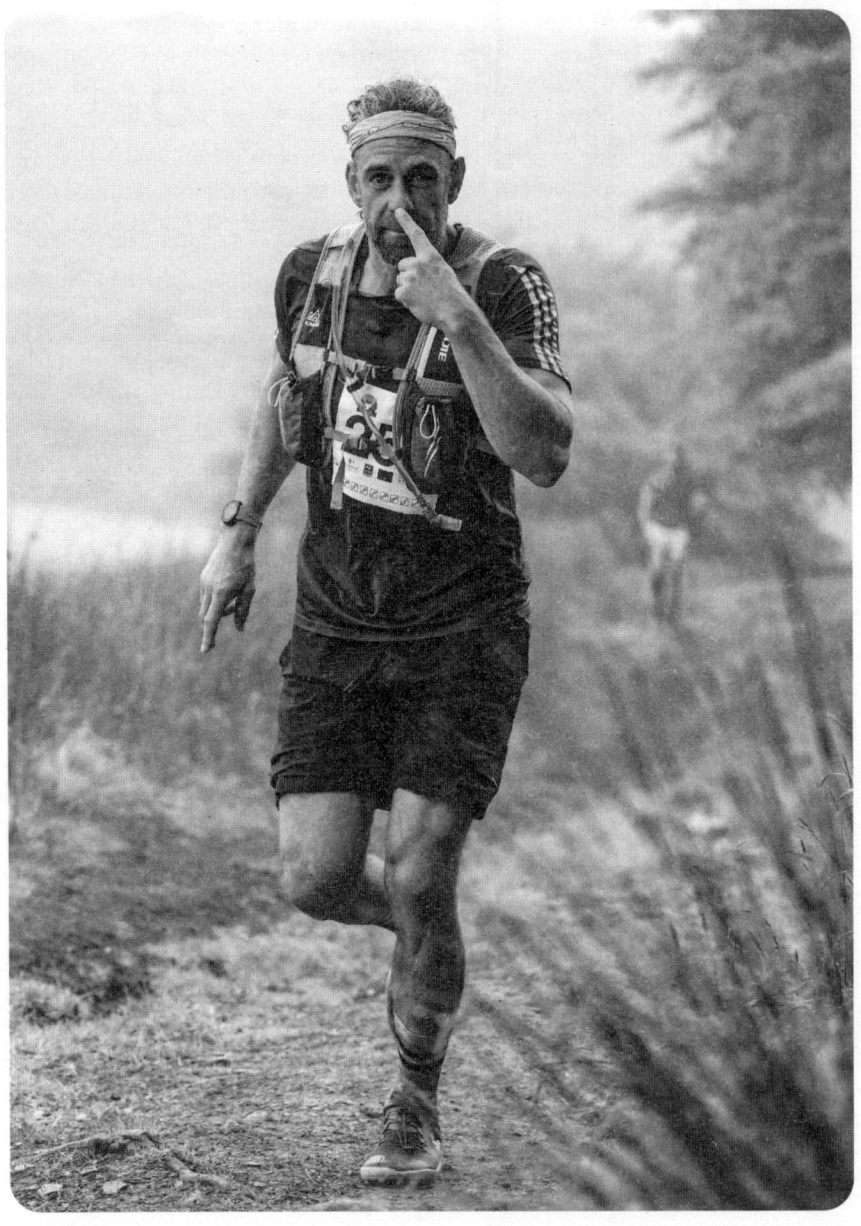